Perspectives on
Long Term
Rehabilitation

How I Achieved a Far Better Recovery from Spinal Cord Injury than Anyone Expected

by
Stacy Holmes

For Lynn

Table of Contents

Perspectives
How I achieved a far better spinal cord injury recovery than anyone expected

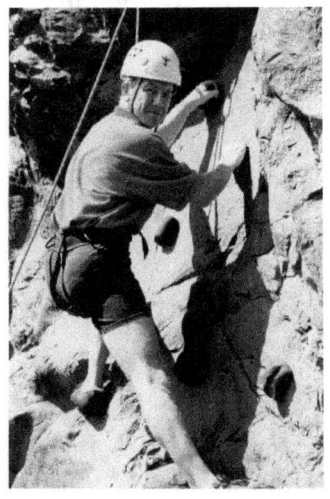

After my first year of life I was walking. I used my biped facility to play baseball with great enthusiasm but little skill. I walked thousands of school hallways and campuses as a student, then teacher, principal and superintendent. I walked out of Walpole (NH) Congregational Church with my new bride Lynn on my arm. I carried my baby daughter Emily. We walked through London's Piccadilly Circus, the Coliseum in Rome, the Eiffel Tower, Costa Rican Indian villages, Denali, Cozumel ruins and many Caribbean beaches. I hiked the Appalachian Trail with my wife, son, brother, niece, nephew and lots of my students and summer campers. And Dad. I walked all over the New England and Arizona trails with Dad.

In my 61st year of life I walked into the neurosurgery pre-op center at Cedars Sinai Medical Center in Los Angeles. I removed my clothes and got into the hospital gown. I laid down on a gurney, never to walk normally again.

In a few hours I awoke from unsuccessful surgery on an intradural melanotic schwannoma at T-11 (about the level of my navel) inside my spinal cord. I was able to use my legs only to wiggle my toes weakly and feebly press my foot down as if on an imaginary car accelerator pedal.

> We must be willing to let go of the life we have planned so as to have the life that is waiting for us.
> **Joseph Conrad**

In the ensuing five years, I progressed from riding a gurney to walking at about 1/3 normal speed for men of my age with a cane and total attention to my jerky barely balancing legs for distances of up to half a mile and durations up to 45 minutes.

This book shares what I, with the many who helped me, did to make a far greater recovery than any physician or physical therapist expected. Some of my physical rehabilitation may have specific relevance only to those with physical disabilities. All of my mental rehabilitation will have relevance to everyone. I write this hoping to give all of you kind enough to visit these pages some valuable insights without your needing to experience paraplegia to discover them.

Notes

All of the internet sites in this book can be reached through http://tinyurl.com/StacyHolmesAuthor. You will not have to type in each site I list in this book. Go to this one site and you can easily click on any site mentioned in this book.

My recovery blog is open to the public at Caringbridge.com/StacyHolmes. I have posted nearly 2000 entries since September 2010. The 37,000 visits to the blog include many comments from friends, family and colleagues that have become part of my story.

The blog is not searchable, but a PDF version of the first 5 years of the blog is searchable. You can find the PDF version at https://drive.google.com/file/d/0B0o-m4Z0IgdTbWVRemZmTzJSUW8/view?usp=sharin

History
Walking to Gurney to Wheelchair to Walker to Crutches to Cane to Walking

The perspectives on disability and rehabilitation offered elsewhere in this book developed during the months before my spinal cord surgery through the following five years. Each chapter is another perspective on that entire period. In contrast to the rest of the book, this chapter travels those years in chronological order. Not many perspectives or insights in this chapter, just the history of what happened.

2010

As the year 2010 began, I was thoroughly enjoying my 40th year in public education. I taught for two years in 1970-2 then launched an administrative career as a principal, a superintendent then a principal again. I started in New

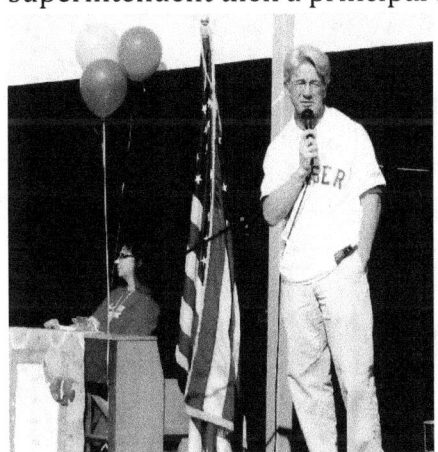

Hampshire, then to Vermont, Massachusetts, New Jersey, New York, Michigan and California. Of all those stops, my last job was best -- principal of a school in Costa Mesa where all the students qualified for free lunch and 95% spoke Spanish as their first language. After 20 years of 10 different timid and often rookie principals, I was the outspoken veteran who finally got the school some respect and a better share of the school district's abundant resources. And fun. The kids, their families and everyone working at Pomona Elementary School enjoyed the experience. "If my health holds out, I'll stay here until I'm 70," I used to say to those asking about my career plans. My health did not hold out.

My wife Lynn had retired from her career in global relocation five years earlier. She concluded her career with Cendant Corporation -- working with Cendant's Fortune 100 clients to manage tax, compensation, relocation and repatriation for their many employees working outside the United States. We were living near three of our eight grand children and enjoying time with them almost daily. Lynn was a Deacon and I was an Elder in our church. We were then and still are officers and board members of Los Niños de la Calle con Wendy charitable foundation.

I had very successful surgery on my right rotator cuff in the late winter and an easy recovery, missing less than a week of work and proceeding pain free through rehabilitation. It would turn out to be remarkable fortune that I elected to have that surgery when I did. A few months later I was depending on my shoulders to support my transfers in and out of wheel chairs, beds, toilets and workout mats when my legs became practically useless.

In the spring, we learned that the Great Recession's devastation of housing prices had recovered enough to make it possible to sell our home in Trabuco Canyon. With our youngest child studying for her doctorate, it was time to admit we were empty nesters with no more need for our 3000-square-foot two-story house. We had no inkling as we tidied up the house for showings that once again our timing was perfect. There is no way our Trabuco Canyon home could have been made handicap accessible, and I was only weeks away from needing an accessible home. Our new home in Mission Viejo was within a few small projects of accessibility. We bought it intending to make it our last home and therefore adaptable to the limitations of our later years. Those limitations came in weeks, not years. We moved just in time.

My spinal cord issues crept in almost unnoticed in those same early months of 2010. I only recognize the first symptoms in retrospect; at the time they did not seem like anything significant. I would scratch at numb spots on my left calf and tug at my sock. It felt like my sock had slipped down when it really had not. I lost the sensation of urine passing so gradually that I cannot really remember when the problem started. By the spring of 2010, though, I could only be sure that I was peeing if I was watching the urine flow. I shrugged it off as just another manifestation of old age. Gray hair, bifocals, deep creases on the face and waning manhood – all part of the passage from middle to old age.

In July the symptoms got suddenly and dramatically much worse. No more shrugging off minor issues and assuming my body was just aging. We visited son Graham and his family in Massachusetts during a July heat wave. My left and right foot got numb. At first the numbness struck just some of the time. But within days I was numb most of the time. The numbness never went above my right ankle, but it traveled up my left leg sometimes as far as my groin. I could still walk and get around all right.

When we got home my family doctor ordered a brain MRI. My sister has multiple sclerosis, so his first concern was MS. The characteristic markers that appear in the brains of MS patients were not there. My family got a chuckle from the radiologist's report that said in part, "...the MRI study of the brain of Mr. Holmes shows nothing remarkable...."

After many inconclusive tests in the neurologist's office, MRIs of the lumbar and then thoracic spine finally revealed an ependymoma about the size of a pencil eraser inside my spinal cord. It had apparently grown enough to interfere with the nerves from my belly button down.

We met with a surgeon in a highly regarded neurosurgery practice near our new home in Mission Viejo. He recommended a procedure that was not high risk surgery, but, in his words, "super high risk surgery." For a second opinion, Lynn managed to wrangle a connection to Keith Black, chief of neurosurgery at Cedars Sinai in Los Angeles. It turned out that Dr. Black only does brain surgery, so we ended up working with his second in command, John Yu. We were impressed with Cedars Sinai and Dr. Yu. We decided to schedule surgery with him.

In retrospect, we should have considered alternatives to surgery. It turned out that my tumor could be killed with a relatively low dose of radiation. My father chose radiation for his prostate cancer, enjoyed a ten-year remission but then a devastating relapse that ended his life in a few excruciating months. He lay near death when he told me never to leave a tumor in my body. "Cut the damn thing out," he told me. With that in mind, I might never have opted for radiation or just watchful waiting instead of surgery anyway.

A retired principal friend was available to substitute for me at my school, which was just starting a new school year. On September 20th Ken took over my school, and I walked normally for the last time in my life into the neurosurgery suite at Cedars Sinai.

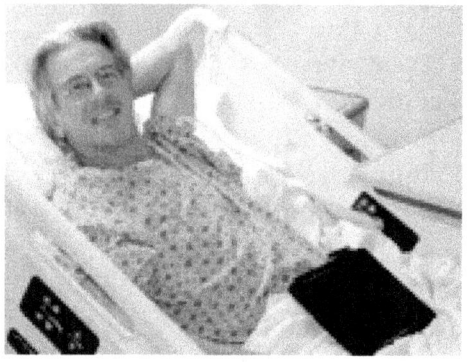 Surgery had to be stopped when it was causing devastating damage to the nerves to my lower body. From the outset, spinal cord surgery caused damage. The laser scalpel severed nerves just opening up my spinal cord. When the tumor was discovered embedded in still more nerves inside the spinal cord, the battle was lost and soon surrendered.

Enough of the tumor was removed to do some pathology studies. The pathologist is 90% certain that it is a melanotic schwannoma. This particular tumor has only been reported in the spinal cords of adults fewer than twenty times. With luck like that, I have stopped buying lottery tickets. Dr. Yu was able to enlarge the space around the tumor in hopes that whatever nerves were still working would have enough space to get around the tumor.

After two days in intensive care and 4 more days in a regular room, I moved to the neurological rehabilitation unit. There I received daily physical and occupational therapy. By the end of the month in the hospital, I could get myself from my bed to my wheel chair. From my wheel chair, I could transfer myself to the toilet, the padded table where I did most of my rehab or the bench I sat on to take my showers. I propelled my wheel chair successfully on a field trip to the shopping mall food court two blocks from the hospital. My bowels and bladder recovered enough sensation that I could feel when I needed to get to the bathroom. That about covered the hospital in-patient rehab goals, at least from the insurance company's perspective.

It was a hectic month for Lynn. I still do not know how she did it. Our new home's front walkway steps became a ramp that looked like the original design. Inside, the front hallway got ramps to the family room and bedrooms, again constructed and stained to look like part of the house, not an add on. Every floor, wall and ceiling was redone. Lynn oversaw all this renovation while never missing a day with me at the hospital, a brutal 90 minutes of southern California driving each way. She also scouted out the options for outpatient rehabilitation, finding the perfect place for me to continue my rehab after leaving the hospital.

> # Work is love made visible.
> ## Kahlil Gibran

I was home in November but back to Cedars Sinai for 5 consecutive day trips getting radiation to kill the tumor. The radiation treatments were an ordeal. I was immobilized in a vest that covered my face, neck and torso. Suffocation and claustrophobia challenged my ability to meditate my way through the sessions. Fortunately, I had none of the indigestion or other side effects common with radiation. I gained the only tattoo on my body – a blue dot in the center of my chest that they used to align the radiation gun. Interestingly, it is nearly the exact spot where a bit of skin cancer appeared four years later.

I started outpatient rehab three days each week. Precision Rehabilitation became my base of recovery for more than four years. My physical therapist was concerned about the leg braces (or AFOs) that I was fitted with at Cedars Sinai. More trips back to Los Angeles to get the braces rebuilt to provide more protection to keep my knees from snapping into a locked position.

I took the first driving lesson of my life at age 62. I had driven farm equipment so much as a teenager that I never took driver education in high school. If you can back up a hay wagon with a tractor, you can parallel park a car. A nice man came to our home one afternoon and showed me the basics of hand control driving. He then had me drive his hand-controlled car for an hour and signed off on my license to drive with hand controls. I drove only short distances on neighborhood streets for a few weeks but was ready to drive the highways by January. No mishaps in the five years of hand control driving since then -- nearly 100,000 miles. I did get rear-ended creeping in heavy traffic, but that was the fault of the lady's cell phone in the car behind me.

Precision Rehabilitation fitted me with a Ti-Lite wheel chair that was custom made to fit my body. Light enough to lift with one hand, it comes apart, so that I can transfer from the wheel chair to the driver's seat of my car, then put the wheel chair in the passenger seat beside me piece by piece.

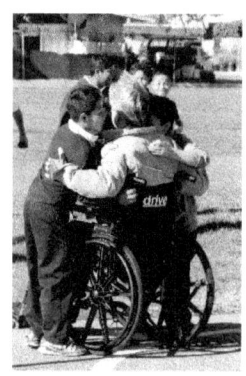

2011
I returned to work in December 2010, catching rides with a principal friend or Lynn. By January, I was driving myself. I went to rehab after work three days each week, then cut back work to only two or three days each week. I could not manage rehab and work on the same day and it became apparent that work would impede my physical recovery. In June 2011 I retired after 40+ years in public education.

In February I took my first steps without a walker. The walker was moved along by an intern, so that it was in front of me if I lost balance. Only a few steps, but an encouraging start.

In March I fell while showering and broke my left fibula (the non weight-bearing bone in my lower leg). No rehab for 3 months. Lynn, who had taught Pilates part-time earlier in her retirement, devised home-bound rehab that kept me moving and getting stronger while leaving my left leg in its Red Sox red cast safely out of the activity. My core and most of my leg muscles actually got stronger while waiting for the fibula to heal. There really is nothing Lynn cannot do.

In July Lynn and I managed a flight to Boston to visit son Graham, wife Jean, daughters Megan and Lauren. Their guest room was up a flight of stairs. I crawled up and down the stairs with anxious family members a step behind me. Using the gangway rails as parallel bars, I supported myself onto a ship to go whale watching outside Boston harbor. With Graham's strong arms helping me transfer into the canoe, I was able to paddle the quiet waters of the upper Charles River. I returned to Fenway Park to see my beloved Red Sox. The 100-year-old park turned out to be amazingly accessible. Those ten days in New England were so encouraging. Travel, family visits and some of my favorite activities were possible once again.

In October I was able to walk a few small steps unassisted (no walker, no cane, no crutches) during rehab sessions with Ziad -- a very strong PT with quick reflexes -- inches away ready to catch me when I lost balance. Holding on to the sides, I walked in son Zachary's backyard pool. I also used an elliptical machine to get some aerobics, strength, balance and walking practice. Zach, his wife Thavy and their children Kyle, Amanda and Emma also live in Mission Viejo, only a few minutes away from us. Their back yard is a water park that provides me with great rehab opportunities.

2012

I have been a lifelong theater lover. Getting back to seeing performances at nearby arts centers was a great step in my recovery. I could wheel chair to the theater seat, transfer and let the usher or Lynn stow the wheel chair out of the way until intermission. I started watching the amateur community theater casting calls and noticed that the Attic Theater in Santa Ana was doing <u>Twelve Angry Men</u>. I auditioned and immediately felt I was

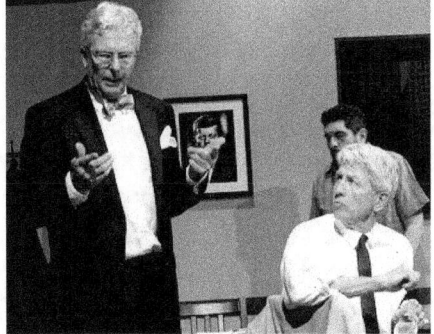

back in the company of great friends, although I knew almost nobody there. When I had trouble stepping up on the stage to audition, another actor came up behind me and said, "You're good. I have your back." With his strong hand between my shoulder blades assuring me I was not going to tumble backwards, I did manage to get both legs and both crutches safely onto the stage.

I played Juror #9, the oldest, who has some nice scenes. Even the small parts are a lot of work in that show, since the entire jury is onstage for the whole play. I used Lofstrand (forearm) crutches to get around on stage.

In June I cut back my rehabilitation sessions to twice each week. About the same time, I started sessions with an acupuncturist. Jun is a gentle Korean with great dedication to his profession. My sessions often ran more than an hour. He started with suctioning and other mechanical stimulation of my circulation. Then he found points from my neck to my buttocks to my ankles to place needles that would encourage nerves to reconnect. After I flipped over, he did more traditional general wellness acupuncture on my arms and legs. I kept seeing him at least weekly until mid-2015.

The Attic Theater invited me back in the fall to direct Pirates of Penzance, the Gilbert and Sullivan operetta. I had last directed adults (in a Gilbert and Sullivan operetta as it happened) in the 1980s when I was a principal in Pequannock Township, NJ. I had a great time with my return to directing. Graduates of opera programs came to the casting call. The music was stunning and the silly slapstick comedy is just what community theater actors and audiences love. Both acting and directing pulled me out multiple times each week, and I struggled to muster enough energy to keep going until 9 or 10 PM for so many nights.

In November my urinary system failed. My prostate had enlarged with age to the point that I could not urinate. I was using a catheter 24/7 for more than a month. My urologist performed my surgery just hours before his break for the Christmas holidays. The catheter came out the day after the transurethral resectioning of my prostate (TURP) procedure. No problems urinating or controlling since then. And none of the dreaded sexual side effects many men have with this surgery. It was nice to have a surgery work out well for a change.

I kept up rehab during the whole urinary ordeal and posted some nice results in the December 2012 progress testing:

- 10-meter unassisted (no cane, no crutches) walk in 28 seconds.
- 7-minute walk on treadmill at 1.3 mph.
- 6-minute walk on crutches at 1.3 mph.
- 45-minute non-stop endurance walk on crutches.

2013

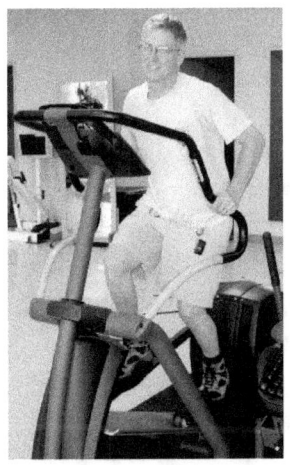

In the following year I directed <u>HMS Pinafore</u>, played Grandpa (the leading role) in <u>You Can't Take It with You</u> and played the Judge in <u>Inherit the Wind</u> at The Attic. I only had to get from the doorway to the judge's bench in <u>Inherit the Wind</u> – an entire show just using a cane.

In July, I cut back my rehabilitation visits to once a week and was able to get to a 24 Hour Fitness gym on my own. A typical workout is over two hours using all the upper body and leg strength machines, doing stretches as well as walking in the swimming pool, on the treadmill and/or in the group exercise room. In the group exercise room I walked for 10-15 minutes, going back and forth next to a dance barre, so there was something to grab when I lost my balance. A few months later, I added side stepping and backward stepping next to the dance barre.

In November, I started using only the cane to get around the house. We removed the ramps and stored the wheel chair in the garage. I did some "furniture walking" without the cane, relying solely on the furniture to catch my balance as I made my way around the house. We also removed the chair in the shower. I started showering standing up, thanking Lynn every time for her ingenious placement of the grab bars in our bathrooms.

2014

I directed <u>One Flew Over the Cuckoo's Nest</u> early in the year. The production was good, something I could be proud of. But some of the undercurrents at the theater were difficult for me. I was happy when the show closed and I took the rest of the year away from The Attic.

In March I had a watershed moment at rehab. Professor Beth Fisher from USC's Division of Biokinesiology and Physical Therapy visited one of the doctoral interns working with me at Precision Rehabilitation. In just a few minutes, Dr. Fisher made dramatic changes in how I was walking. The walking on my heels with my butt sticking out was finally addressed in a way I could understand. She suggested some moves to focus on while walking that gave me much more forward momentum and got me off my heels.

I walked half a mile on crutches in less than 20 minutes for the first time and began walking around the house unassisted all the time. The cane stayed in the car. I used the cane for trips to the store and the mobility scooter for distances of more than half a mile or durations more than half an hour. The cartilage in my thumbs wore out with the years of wheel chair pushing and crutch walking, so I began to see a thumb specialist every three or four months. Cortisone shots relieve the pain for a few weeks at a time, but the doctor sees surgery as inevitable. I need both my hands to bathe, drive and get around the house safely; I cannot imagine even a few weeks of post-surgical healing and rehab without the use of one of my hands.

In the periodic assessments in the clinic the numbers were improving. Two years back some of my tests showed:
- 10-meter unassisted walk in 28 seconds.
- 7-minute walk on treadmill at 1.3 mph.
- 6-minute walk on crutches at 1.3 miles.
- 45-minute non-stop endurance walk on crutches.

By the end of 2014,
- 10-meter unassisted walk in 18 seconds
- 10 -15 minutes on treadmill at 2.1 mph and 2% incline
- 6-minute walk at the same speed but accomplished on just a cane
- 45 minutes was still about my limit for non-stop endurance walks.

In December I walked to the corner of our street and back just holding Lynn's hand. Neither of us thought we would ever walk down the street holding hands again. One of those small moments with a big impact.

2015

Now in my 4th year of active rehabilitation, I look back months or even years to gauge progress. At the community center down the hill from our home is a walkway with an optional loop that is either half a mile or three quarters of a mile accordingly with only gentle rises and declines. I made a half-mile walk using just my cane for the first time in January.

January through March, Lynn and I collaborated on The Mikado at The Attic Theater. She was assistant director/ assistant costumer / props master and much more. It was much better than spending so many nights apart when I am doing a show. Once again we attracted many great operatic voices that normally do not come out for auditions at The Attic. It was an amazing show. Great performers are not always great people off stage, but this cast was a fun group.

I spent much of this year tinkering with my medication. I had been on Baclofen since 2011 and I had pretty much denied the pain, jerks and intense cramps especially at the end of the day that the Baclofen did not prevent. All my workouts and rehab made my muscles stronger and therefore now capable of much more powerful spasms and cramps. I researched the remarkable improvements marijuana accomplished for pediatric epileptics and adult MS patients. I tracked down some of the same forms of marijuana used with MS patients and epileptics. I was not impressed with the results and it seemed to depress my libido. I tried Gabapentin and Zanaflex, the only FDA approved drugs for spasticity. Zanaflex makes me too foggy to drive a car. By year's end I was back on just Baclofen again, same dose as before, with half the dose of Gabapentin than was originally prescribed. With those I also use Valtoran, a topical NSAID gel, to get some relief from sharp pains in my hip flexors. Once a month or so I take a Norco (Acetaminophen and Hydrocodone) if the pain is keeping me from sleeping.

Dr. Ziad Dahdul, the PT who managed most of my first four years of outpatient rehabilitation left to join a different PT clinic. It was time to spend more time rehabbing and less time commuting. One of the USC doctoral interns asked me if I knew about Complete Balance Solutions, a PT clinic much closer our home in Mission Viejo. I decided to check it out.

Complete Balance Solutions gave me the fresh start I needed. Complete Balance, as you might guess from the name, focuses on balance. They measure the extent to which my visual, inner ear and proprioceptive (touch) systems contribute to my balance. My great weakness is proprioception. I do not know where my feet are unless I am looking at them. I cannot feel whether my toe is pointed straight ahead or sideways, for example.

My new PT, Dr. Mary Beth Pongetti, is the most academically accomplished PT I have ever met. With post-doctoral specialist certifications in neurological and orthopedic disabilities as well as certification as a strength trainer, she has mastered all the book learning and synthesized it into practice during her years at Complete Balance. She has identified my left leg as the weak partner in my walking and my gluts as the non-performers in the musculature necessary to walk faster and steadier. She challenges my balance with a specialized machine that makes the walls and floor move while I try to keep my balance. I also do a series of activities with my eyes closed to force my proprioception and inner ear to hold my balance without any visual assistance. In 2010, if I closed my eyes while standing, I did not know if I was upright or sideways; five years later, my body has figured out ways to use the nerves that still work to tell me I am leaning right or left, forward or backward, although still not fast enough or accurately enough to allow me to stand with my eyes closed washing my face at the bathroom sink for more than a couple seconds.

We flew to Boston then drove to Maine with son Graham, wife Jean, and their daughters Megan and Lauren for a week in Tenant's Harbor. I managed to get into a kayak with Graham's help and enjoy the protected coves and inlets of the rugged Atlantic shoreline. I practiced my walking around the large lawn at the rental house and managed the stairs up to our bedroom unassisted (thanks to two sturdy banisters).

We were already into the next show at The Attic when we left for our Maine vacation. I was casting and doing script work on the trip. When we were already a week into rehearsals the Attic lost the rights to do <u>Guys and Dolls</u> because a professional touring company scheduled a stop in Los Angeles to perform the show. We scrambled to recast the actors and actresses in <u>A Funny Thing Happened on the Way to the Forum</u>, the replacement show. We returned home to discover the costumer had plans to travel in Utah during the two weeks we needed to get the cast costumed as ancient Romans. Lynn rescued the show by designing and sewing wonderful costumes from fabrics she bargained for at nearby swap meets. I was able to handle four-hour rehearsals, getting up on my feet much of the time to walk between two rows of theater seats using the seat backs for balance. We had another successful production with a friendly, talented cast, but we were exhausted after the run of the show.

There was no down time between projects. Lynn had secured a grant from the local water company to replace the turf in our front and back yards to reduce water consumption. The project had to be done by November to be eligible for funding. I was able to do a lot of the heavy work loading and unloading dozens of bags of soil, mulch, sand and fertilizer from Lynn's Jeep. We had larger loads of pea stone and decomposed granite dumped in our driveway. I managed wheelbarrow and lawn-cart loads from the driveway to the front and back yards. Lynn picked out individual decorative stones as carefully as she would choose new clothes for a grandchild. I carried them from the Jeep to their final placements. The raised beds in the back yard required some work swinging a pick-ax, maneuvering the large wooden frames of the raised beds and spreading landscape fabric. We had a crew help us for three weekends, but we kept the projects going on our own during the weeks in between. My strength, balance and endurance had their biggest challenge since my surgery for that month of heavy yard work. If we thought we were tired after the show, we were really tired after the turf removal project!

Thanksgiving was the beginning of a quieter, more restful month for us, albeit clouded with Lynn's impending surgeries in early 2016 for stenosis in her cervical spine and fusing two vertebrae in her lumbar spine. With hand controls in the Jeep installed this year, we had a better riding, roomier car to visit daughter Emily and fiancé Steve's home in Sacramento. Steve is finishing his degree in food science at UC Davis this year. Dr. Emily is in her second year of practice after completing veterinary college in 2014.

       I am grateful to find the motivation to work out at the gym twice a week and to rehab at Complete Balance twice a week as well. More than five years into rehabilitation, it feels like I have the best schedule of independent gym sessions and PT clinic sessions ever.

Notes

The story of another man's recovery from spinal cord tumor surgery is beautifully written in Reynolds Price's, <u>A Whole New Life</u>. Amazon has it as a book or electronic book.

The Attic Theater is at OCAct.com. A clip from my acting as Grandpa in You Can't Take it With You is at
https://www.youtube.com/watch?v=fkTqeJ7TysQ
A trailer-style of clips from Funny Thing Happened on the Way to the Forum is at www.youtube.com/watch?v=kIMDfzABQFU

Kayaking in Maine video:
https://www.youtube.com/watch?v=O1zHUP4q5mw

More on the way the body's three balance systems work is available at <u>http://vestibular.org/understanding-vestibular-disorder/human-balance-system</u>

A short homemade video of the turf removal project is at
<u>https://www.youtube.com/watch?v=l8ob9tkOxb0</u>

Remember, all of the internet sites in this book can be reached through <u>http://tinyurl.com/StacyHolmesAuthor</u>.

Seven Deadly Sins
How I have sinned to help my recovery

Somewhere in the Dark Ages, a group of ascetic monks in Egypt developed a list of seven bad thoughts that a good Christian must overcome. By 400 AD the list had made it to Europe. "The Seven Deadly Sins" was popularized by writings and artwork. The Roman Catholic Church took up the list for use in religious education and confession.

I'm not Catholic but I have heard of the seven deadly sins from time to time since middle school. In some odd moments over the first five years of my rehabilitation, I thought of each of these seven deadly sins with an ironic twist. Each "sin" in its own way has helped me keep going, enjoy life and get better:

- Gluttony
- Lust
- Greed
- Pride
- Sorrow
- Anger
- Sloth.

Gluttony

I have always struggled to keep my weight up. I know, not too many people sympathize with my problem. Within a few days after my spinal cord surgery, nurses and doctors started clucking about my weight loss. I could not figure out how they knew, but it turns out the fancy beds in hospitals also measure how heavy the patient is. Tricky. I pretty much ate as much as I wanted of whatever I wanted before the tumor. After surgery, with very little physical activity to stimulate my appetite, I had to work harder to get my weight back. Another irony. Most people gain weight when they are inactive. I lose my appetite.

The hospital food service started bringing me cake at 10 PM in addition to the regular 3 meals. Lynn brought me Boost Plus, a 360-calorie meal replacement, starting the habit that I continue today of drinking a meal replacement shake in the middle of the night. When I wake up to use the bathroom, I drink a shake. I got back over 160 pounds and have hovered around 165 ever since.

My cholesterol is not what one would expect for a lean guy who works out 4 times a week, but it is not horrible either. So I continue to enjoy premium ice cream before turning in for bed. Rehab friends of mine often have more regimented diets than I do. But one of the delightful sins we all share is indulgence, whether it is comfort food, chocolate, marijuana or booze.

For me, gluttony is that escape from disability I so often long for. I am not crippled when I am slurping down 3 scoops of ice cream, with fancy hot fudge from the microwave and a waffle cookie on the side. I'm just a kid enjoying a treat without a care in the world.

Lust

My tumor is at T-11, the last vertebra in the mid-spine or thoracic region. Everything south of my belly button has to send and receive messages around the tumor and through the area scorched by the surgeon's laser scalpel. Many messages never make it to the brain going up; many commands never make it down.

During my surgery, Dr. Yu came out to speak with Lynn to tell her I was paralyzed and most of the tumor was still in me. Somehow she withstood that news and kept hoping. I will never know how. According to the surgeon, every nerve below the tumor was cut off – literally. Later, as I emerged from anesthesia, someone told me to wiggle my toes and I did. The surgeon returned to Lynn with better news. Attempting to remove the tumor had done terrible damage, but some nerves were still intact.

In the next month of hospitalization, they gathered extensive data about the nerves in my lower body – mapping what I could feel and which reflexes still functioned. I got lots of questions about my urination and defecation. After all, as soon as the basic waste channels are working again, most insurance companies think it is time for the patient to go home.

Sex was conspicuously omitted from the many questions or physical probes. They touched me almost all over with pins to map where my nerves still worked well enough to have light touch sensation. Almost, that is. No tests of the penis, scrotum or anus. They asked me if I could feel when I needed to pee or poop, if I could feel waste leaving my body and many more yucky questions. But no questions about sexual sensation, erections or ejaculations.

So I broke the silence about 2 weeks after the surgery when one of the chief rehab doctors stopped by on evening rounds. Intending just to poke his head in and move on, Dr. Rau pulled up a chair and chatted for a few minutes after I asked my question. He said lots of nerves recover in the first year after a spinal cord injury and things that I could not feel a month after surgery might recover in time. Or not. No one could predict which nerves will function again, how well or when. In a year and a half, he said, there probably would not be any more nerves recovering.

More than five years after the surgery, I still have considerable loss of sexual sensation that now appears to be permanent. Men are aroused and achieve psychogenic erections (from the brain) by non-touch stimulation, e.g. seeing a naked person or sexual thoughts. The brain has to have working nerve connections with the genitals for that to work. I have lost a lot of that kind of arousal. Fortunately for me, men also get reflex erections that do not originate in the brain. These erections are stimulated by touch that triggers a reflex in my sacral spine (the lowest region of the spine). Strangely, my brain my not be aware the touch is happening but the reflex works because it only has to travel from my genitals to the nearby sacral spine and back again. Even though my brain is not enjoying the whole event, I achieve erections and orgasms. What I do feel I gratefully savor and enjoy. I have more sexual function than many, probably most, spinal cord injury patients.

And I was close to assuming sex was all gone after the surgery, judging by the silence of the doctors. The lesson: keep in *touch* with the sin of lust. Break the silence with the rehabilitation doctors. There are drugs, prostheses, toys and techniques to explore.

Four complete SCI (severed spinal cord) men in a UCLA study were implanted with electric probes. They were able to stand for the first time since their injuries when the electrodes were turned on. An unexpected side effect was the return of their sexual functions. One became a father.

In the movie The Intouchables (based on a true story), a quadriplegic hires a beautiful call girl to massage his ear lobes, the only place on his body where he can still feel something sensual.

We get around differently after a spinal cord injury, but we still get around. So we may be sexual men and women differently after SCI, but we remain sexual nevertheless.

Greed

"He who dies with the most toys, wins." This was on the sweatshirt of a young CPA in my class at Rutgers Law School. Already married with kids and more than 15 years into my career in public school administration, I was one of few older students going to law school at night. I sat in front of toys-boy with his brazen sweatshirt, so I overheard his marriage plans as he chatted with his buddy. I would love to know how the marriage worked out. He was so adamant that his new wife would have to let him have his toys. He was maybe thirty years old and apparently a fast-rising accountant about to acquire a wife, perhaps to round out his collection that included a hot car, motorcycle, jet ski, snow mobile, boat, ATV and probably much more.

My greed for toys has given my rehabilitation from spinal cord injury a new focus several times over the past 5 years. An upcoming chapter describes how each device helped me physically, but the mere acquisition was a delightful sin. My Ti-Lite wheel chair is red with front wheels that flash colored lights as they roll, just like the fancy sneakers lucky little kids get from Santa. I concocted a rationale for the insurance company that the colors made me more approachable for my students at school;

insurance paid the extra costs for the wheels and the red frame. Persuading the insurance people was almost as fun as riding in the red wheel chair with blinking front wheels.

I did not need the wheel chair after a few years, and it is now stored in our garage. But I still need my mobility scooter to manage shopping malls, airports and any walking beyond half a mile or half an hour. It is red as well, of course, and I can load it into the back of my Prius by myself. It comes apart in 5 pieces, each light enough to lift with one hand. I enjoy the attention I get at the mall when I use the car for support to get to the hatchback, take out the scooter pieces, put them together, and buzz off to people watch and window shop. Or maybe even buy something.

We have installed hand controls in both our cars, so that I can drive our old Prius or our very old Jeep -- an extravagance I have not second-guessed for a moment. Finding devices that will help me and indulging in them has been a thoroughly enjoyable greed. Getting insurance companies to pay at least their fair share has been a challenge; each victory a gratifying success.

We have Direct TV feeds at each of our desks in the office and in the combination guest room/ sewing room / play room, as well as the main set up in the family room. I have to stop a few times every day. Recordings of all our favorite shows are waiting to make those breaks more enjoyable. Games on a cool cell phone, a book to read on a Kindle or to a book to write on my laptop have added to my greedy collection of toys.

I don't drool over the ads for high tech gear to go hiking in the mountains anymore. I gave away all my fancy office furniture, books and art when I took disability retirement from public education. Now I keep up with websites and magazines where I might find a faster mobility scooter or a phone that will compensate for my aging memory.

Greed is a pro-active sin. I don't wait for a doctor or therapist to suggest a new pill or gadget. I find out everything that SCI patients are using and ask my physician or physical therapist if any of them might help me. I am greedily gathering in all the toys of disability, to be sure. But it is another life function that can keep going even after disability: Good old American acquiring more and more stuff. A sinful way to stay informed about the options for happiness and a better rehabilitation.

Pride

I have kept a blog going on Caring Bridge since my diagnosis with a spinal cord tumor in 2010. For the first years my posts were daily, now once or twice a month. I range into political rants and reviews of books and movies, but the center focus is the progress of my rehabilitation. Here is where the sin of pride shines brightest. I chronicle each bit of progress. How long it takes me to walk a half-mile on my crutches, for example. Or the results of a push-ups contest after dinner with grandson Kyle and stepson Zach (I won). Anything I do that I can count, time or measure becomes a point of pride. I post my personal bests, breakthroughs and improvements.

But there is also a dark side to manage. I look at people walking on the sidewalk with no problems keeping their balance and grumble. For all the "progress" I cheer about, I still can't simply walk down the street like all those people do. I never realized getting off a gurney and walking again required so many levels of progress. Each improvement seems barely to nudge me closer to my ultimate goals. There's no denying I'm doing better than a year ago, but there is also no denying I am still not walking like other people.

> I would rather laugh with the sinners than cry with the saints.
>
> Billy Joel

Seeing friends or family from out of town bolsters my pride. The progress I sometimes do not recognize from day to day or week to week, they do notice from one occasional visit to the next. Even the PT who fills in when Mary Beth has to miss one of my sessions boosts my pride when she tells me how much better I am doing since the last time we worked together.

I take pride in my appearance, my community theater work, how much I can help with housework and gardening, my piano playing, writing and gaming (Sudoku, bridge, Lumosity). Some activities I do as well as or even better than I could before my disability. Most get better or at least easier for me to do with practice.

Most of the 67-year-old guys at the gym are trying to do the same workout they did when they were 66 years old and are not succeeding. I'm doing more at 67 than I could at 66. Pride – a wonderfully motivational sin.

Sorrow

Cedars-Sinai Medical Center wisely staffed the neurological rehab unit with a psychologist, a nice guy who visited me a few times and then said he would just come by once in a while after that. He pronounced me well-adjusted and accepting of my disability. We both had spent time in Michigan and enjoyed each other's repartee about Michigan, psychology, medicine and the bizarre political campaign that was in its final stages at the time (two CEOs with no background in public service were trying to buy the governorship and one of the US Senate seats in California – they failed).

Notwithstanding the psychologist's appraisal, I did have my moments of sorrow, but mostly after midnight. The limited hospital TV programming was down to late night reruns, Jay Leno, and CNN's repeating the same news they had broadcast all day. Lynn had gone home, and the hospital staff came by only to dump out my urinal once or twice for the rest of the night.

I called these late night mental collapses "demons." The silence of the late night alone in my hospital room invited demons who would tell me I would never work again, never hike the Appalachian Trail again, never walk, never be able to take care of myself, and on and on. Never this, never that.

My sanity was preserved by my lifelong ability to fall asleep quickly and so deeply that I rarely remember my dreams. Siblings, college roommates, and Lynn have heard me dreaming and talking in my sleep all my life. But I remember nothing. So the demons would gather as I turned off the TV and got settled for the night. They had to work fast because I would drop off to sleep within a few minutes. The next morning they had to retreat to the back of my mind as I attended to my new life of rehab, learning to get to the bathroom on spastic legs and otherwise how to use the nerves that still worked to do the work of others that were gone.

When I confronted the reality a few months later that I could not both work as a school principal and do all the needed rehab, I let go of the profession I loved. I had planned to work until I was 70, but my body would not go where my spirit was headed. The good-byes with colleagues were not too hard; I knew I would keep in touch with a few of them, and I have. But seeing the students on the playground for the last time, visiting classrooms and presenting awards at our monthly celebrations – those were sad partings. I am frequently amazed at how remote the memory of a 40-year career has become. I vividly remember things that happened and cannot believe I actually was there, in charge and doing all that I did. It is almost like I am watching someone else living my life on TV or in a book.

Lynn and I both had high-powered careers. She spent years as a Senior Vice President at Prudential traveling most of the time to clients all over the country. I was busy with school board meetings and graduate school studies late into the night two or three times each week for almost all of my 40 years in school leadership. We were working full time, raising a family full time and catching up with each other on Sunday mornings and vacations. Lynn retired a few years before my tumor showed up; so when I had to retire, we were suddenly together all day every day for the first time in more than 30 years. As I saw my last day of work approaching, I recalled the wry joke one of my teachers shared when I asked her if she was going to retire now that her husband had retired. "Nope," she said, "I married him for better or for worse, but not for lunch."

Fortunately, Lynn and I thoroughly enjoy lunches together and our marriage has come into its best years now that neither of us has a job to pull us apart. We still have separate interests and activities. We are both fortunate to be so independent. We also have many projects that we undertake together and an abundance of shared entertainment and fun. As one cherished relationship, activity or project comes to an end, that end has made another beginning possible. My career ended prematurely; our marriage flourished as never before.

Seven Deadly Sins: *How sin helps recovery*

I do not think I deny or fail to notice what I have lost, but like the demons in the hospital, the losses cannot capture the spirit of a man who has already moved to a new life that does not depend upon running a school, hiking the Appalachian Trail or even walking. My life as a walking person is a series of grateful, not sorrowful, memories. I am grateful that I did so much with the gifts I had for the time I had them. Lynn and I saw Paris when we could both walk the beautiful boulevards. I hiked with Dad when he was still alive. And a few thousand kids read better and enjoy learning more because I ran their school or their school's district.

I love musical theater, and so it is natural for me to hear a tune and recall a lyric when I try to understand life. In the musical Chorus Line, an aspiring dancer about to break through and win a

> Kiss today good-bye and point me towards tomorrow…
> from Chorus Line

role in a Broadway show falls and fractures her ankle, a career ending injury for a show dancer. As they help her from the stage, she sings, "Kiss today goodbye and point me toward tomorrow…." And later, "Look, my eyes are dry. The gift was ours to borrow…."

Indeed, all that we have in life is never forever ours, or even ours for the rest of today. We can do good work, help others, love, laugh and – yes – walk for this moment only. Even those who can walk normally are only temporarily able bodied. So, rather than grieve for what we have lost, it's best to take a loss as a reminder that what we still have is guaranteed only for the next moment. It is always time to make the most of what we still have.

Anger

When my older brother was in first grade and I was an infant, he drew a picture of me in school. His teacher asked why he drew his brother's face all red. "He's always screaming," Ed explained. A nurse dropped me when I was four days old and broke my arm. I don't know how the first three days of my life went, but I complained about my arm strapped in a splint enough to keep

25

my face red much of the time after that. I have been easily angered ever since. My frequent fits of rage earned me the nickname "Fitsy" from my older brother and sister.

I was battling a big hospital and a bigger insurance company during most of my month at Cedars-Sinai Medical Center. My surgeon visited me in the days after surgery and said I was going to the rehab ward. The hospital and insurance company took another week before I was actually on the rehab unit. In one of my calls to my insurance company to negotiate how long I could stay on the rehab unit, I discovered the insurance company actually had a nurse with an office directly overseeing the company's cases at Cedars-Sinai. I got myself in my wheelchair and headed out into the hallway. The nurses were pleased that I was getting a little exercise. I zipped down the hall to the elevator and popped down to the Anthem insurance lady's office. Without her customary insulation of staff and telephone, she decided to come to an agreement with an angry old guy in pajamas.

My family and therapists hear me scolding my legs as I try to move them all the time. Much of my rehabilitation is motivated by my angry battle against a spastic uncomfortable body. Rather than submit to the cramps my legs get after hours of nerve spasms, I do a long series of stretches on the floor or get up on my legs and walk for half an hour to tire out the muscles that are hurting me. Even if my legs are so bad that my crutches / walker / cane is carrying most of the load, I fight back. I argue with my legs. I refuse to let my messed-up nerves win.

Sloth

My sister Nancy has had multiple sclerosis for more than 20 years. She offers good advice on balancing activities. Disability is a long haul, if you are lucky. It can shorten the life of the disabled person who burns out after a few months of intense but ultimately frustrating rehabilitation. Even the weekend warrior style of rehabilitation may shorten life. That is, a huge workout followed by two or more days of nothing. With MS, SCI or other disabilities, days of doing nothing physically or mentally take a greater toll, as do days of doing too much. The trick is consistency and moderation.

When I had just begun to have enough energy to go see a play at a nearby theater, my legs would be so tired by that time of day that they would jerk and tremble while I was just sitting still. I had to explain to the person seated next to me that one or both legs might start to move later in the performance. I took it as a breakthrough when I could sit and watch an evening performance without jerking legs.

For more than 5 years of rehabilitation, my sin of sloth has helped sustain my steady pace of rehabilitation. I often take a day off to play familiar, easy pieces on the piano instead of studying the difficult new piece for my next lesson. I play easier games on my phone when I do not feel like concentrating on a hard one. I take a day off from exercise after a two-hour session in the gym. Not as intense a regimen as one might expect of the diligent piano student, rehabilitating paraplegic or dedicated gamer. But then, I am still enjoying piano, rehabbing enough to accomplish consistent improvement and keeping my retired brain sharp. I owe the improvements to hard work; I owe the long-term consistent effort as much to my shamelessly sinful sloth as my work ethic.

Summary
Frequent sinning has helped my rehabilitation. I am – in my own way -- gluttonous, lustful, greedy, proud, sorrowful, angry and slothful. And, I am happier, more active and more optimistic as a result. It is hard being disabled and hard to be virtuous. So cut yourself a little slack on the virtuous life and perhaps you will make steadier progress with your disabilities.

Notes
Enabling Romance is a book written to guide disabled persons to regain their sex lives.

A list of seven heavenly virtues, to oppose the seven deadly sins, appeared in an epic poem entitled *Psychomachia*, or *Battle/Contest of the Soul*. Written by Aurelius Clemens

Seven Deadly Sins: *How sin helps recovery*

Prudentius, a Christian governor who died around 410 A.D. The virtues are identified as chastity, temperance, charity, diligence, patience, kindness, and humility. Practicing them is said to protect one against temptation from the seven deadly sins. In the musical Camelot, Mordred declares these virtues as "deadly" and therefore not part of his life.

You can hear the song at
https://www.youtube.com/watch?v=AT3x2yi05Hs

Intouchables
After an accident leaves him a quadriplegic, a denizen of France's high society hires a young man from the ghetto to serve as his caretaker. Trailer:
https://www.youtube.com/watch?v=34WIbmXkewU

The Sessions Fox Searchlight
A young man in an iron lung seeks the assistance of a sex surrogate. A Sundance Film Festival winner. Trailer:
https://www.youtube.com/watch?v=Fy2y7UIpgP4

Sex after a spinal cord injury is discussed from a medical perspective by doctors and nurses at
http://www.facingdisability.com/expert-topics/sex-and-fertility-after-sci is a useful site for a number of other topics as well.

The UCLA study of quadriplegics and paraplegics regaining sexual function with electrical stimulation is well reported in New Mobility: http://www.newmobility.com/2016/02/epi-stim/

Remember, all of the internet sites in this book can be reached through http://tinyurl.com/StacyHolmesAuthor. You will not have to type in each site I like in the book. Go to this one site and you can easily click on any site mentioned in this book.

Devices
How a succession of devices advanced my rehabilitation

More than a dozen mobility devices, electronics and gadgets were prescribed for me in the five years after my spinal cord tumor surgery. My doctors and therapists thought some of them were my final plateau. I would hear statements like, "Now you can get your wheelchair in and out of the car by yourself." Or, "Well that's good. You can get around on crutches now." But I never saw my wheelchair, walker or crutches as a final solution. Eager as I was to get to the next device, as soon as I was using it I started looking forward to the day I would no longer need it.

I was and still am powerfully motivated to get to the next device, believing that one day it will be *no* device. Some electronics and gadgets did not have such an obvious progression, but caught my interest as possible silver bullets. With drugs, acupuncture and electronics, I always hope they will wake up all the dead nerves and splice all the broken connections. So far, nothing has been the drug or device to make me dramatically better overnight. But like the little kid in the old joke, I keep digging through the manure sure I will one day find my pony.

Sometimes epic insurance company battles have been necessary to get the funds to pay for one of these gizmos. Other times, I was all ready to go to war then my insurance company would pay without a problem. Horizon Blue Cross Blue Shield of NJ has proven to be a great supplement to Medicare.

So here goes, the devices presented roughly in order of appearance:

AFO Leg Braces

AFO (ankle foot orthosis) braces were prescribed for me while I was 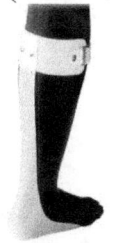 still in the hospital. A technician made a plaster mold of my foot (quite a messy procedure) then a plastic brace was made from that mold. The AFOs were prescribed to keep my knees from locking. My muscles were so atrophied and out of control that my knees would snap into a hyperextension. When the AFOs had to be remade to suit the specifications of my outpatient rehabilitation, Lynn and I got to meet a great character and craftsman. Max has been fabricating prosthetic limbs and all manner of braces for decades. His devices, unique for each patient, are works of art. His stories and humor each time we met created memories that I will always revisit with a smile.

I wore the AFOs every day for many months. They kept my knees from locking, but got in the way of so many of the exercises I was doing at rehabilitation that I stopped wearing them. I expected the PTs to notice and tell me to keep wearing them, but nobody ever said anything. Perhaps my control of my knees had improved enough to make the AFOs optional.

The AFOs' influence on my gait did not go away so easily. The AFOs prevented me from locking my knees for the first year or more that I was struggling to stand and take a few steps leaning heavily on a walker. Not being able to straighten my knees with the AFOs on, I could not get my weight on my toes nor could I get my legs lined up hip to knee to ankle the way normal people do. For at least the next four years after wearing the AFOs, I was working to get my weight to land on my heel, roll forward onto my toe and then push off from the toe as my weight shifted to the other foot. Even with the support of a walker or crutches, it was a battle. I have also been struggling to get my butt to stop sticking out and walk fully upright. Without some kind of protection, perhaps my knees would have been injured before I had enough strength and control to keep them from snapping into hyperextension. I just wish someone had told me the AFOs were saving my knees at the expense of my gait. It would have helped me focus better on what needed to be fixed when I was able to stop using the AFOs.

I put the AFOs on and walked for a few yards in 2016, four years since the last time I wore them. I was amazed at how confining they were. I gave myself retroactive extra credit for all that I achieved while wearing the AFOs. After the surgery wiped out control and sensation in my legs with significant muscle atrophy, I then tried to get the little muscle I had left to hold me up between spasms. And just to make sure that was not too easy, I strapped on AFOs that kept my knees from straightening.

Devices: *How a succession of devices advanced my rehabilitation*

FES Bike

Restorative Technologies makes a series of products to reprogram nerves as well as build strength and endurance. Within my first month or two of outpatient rehabilitation, I started sessions on the FES (functional electrical stimulation) bike. Electrodes attach to muscles needed to pedal the bike. Once the electrodes are in place and the patient's feet are strapped onto the pedals of the bike, the unit zaps the muscles in the sequence and pattern necessary to make the legs pedal the bike. The software senses when the patient is pedaling on his/her own and backs off the zapping. Just getting legs to do any patterned movement again is helpful. Working muscles to rebuild strength is hard when you cannot make your legs do anything; the bike gets the muscles working again whether they can manage the pedaling motion independently or not.

In 2011, during the first six months after surgery, I was trying to do rehab after working all day at school. I would get so tired that I would fall asleep on the FES bike. The clinic started giving me a pillow to rest my head on as I dozed and the FES bike kept my legs pumping for half an hour. It was a funny sight, and one of the events that convinced me to apply for disability retirement and stop trying to combine rehab with the responsibilities of a school principal.

Walker

The walker was in my life starting in the hospital. At first, I would support my weight with my hands on the walker enough to slide a foot forward. You could not really call it a step, but I could lift my weight off my feet enough with my hands to slide a weightless foot forward. A nurse's aide would be behind me with a wheelchair to catch me if I lost balance or got so worn out that I could not make my feet slide forward anymore. Later, when I was using crutches for most of my stops at stores and offices, I still used the walker for the riskier walking, such as the gym's wet pool deck.

At first my gait was so wide I kicked the legs of the walker. A year later, my gait had narrowed so that I stayed well within the perimeter of the walker's legs. On the down side, walkers encourage leaning forward and hunching shoulders – more bad habits to correct as the walker was phased out and the crutches replaced it.

Dashaway

Traditional walkers are wonderfully supportive. I rarely feel so secure as I do using a walker. But their design makes it too easy to hunch forward and look down while walking. Stanley Dashew, an inventor who lived from 1916 to 2013 and is best known for inventing the embossing machine that made the plastic credit card

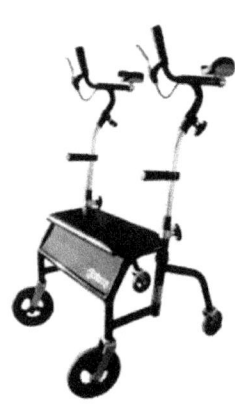

possible, improved the walker by inventing the Dashaway late in his remarkable life. The frame of the Dashaway is much higher (and adjustable) so that you stand fully upright to walk with it. Instead of leaning on your hands, your entire forearms rest on padded supports and your hands only work the brakes. It even has a padded shelf about knee high, so that the patient can stop and take a seat once in a while. The brakes can be set up so that the Dashaway only rolls when the patient is squeezing the brake handles open, or the brakes can work in just the opposite manner and stop the Dashaway when the patient squeezes the handles.

The Dashaway was my first solo walking. I would get to rehabilitation early, change clothes, do my stretches then walk around the clinic on my own with the Dashaway until my PT session started. I advocated the Dashaway to my sister Nancy who suffers from MS. She has used it for mobility around her neighborhood, home and her current assisted living home. She relies mostly on her motorized wheelchair now, but still gets some exercise on the Dashaway.

Ti-Lite Wheelchair

I went through a succession of wheelchairs. In the hospital I plopped into whatever wheelchair was handy. I learned to drive these large, heavy wheel chairs around the hospital. I mastered stopping, cornering and backing. Setting brakes before getting into or out of the chair became a safety habit. I was discharged from the hospital with a new but still standard issue chair. Not quite as heavy or wide as the hospital chairs, but still a two-handed heave into the back of the car for Lynn (and later me).

Devices: *How a succession of devices advanced my rehabilitation*

At outpatient rehab I acquired a Ti-Lite wheel chair. Made of aircraft aluminum (a even lighter titanium alloy is available) I could lift the whole chair with one hand. Once I was able to drive myself with hand controls I could disassemble the wheelchair and stow it in the passenger seat beside me.

Wheelchair seating is an advanced skill, and I was fortunate to have a PT with more than a decade of experience taking more measurements than a tailor needs to fit me with a fine set of custom-made clothes. The fit is more than just measurements, however. Christy made choices that I could not have made for myself, and the wheelchair salesman would have just defaulted to what most people choose. For example, Christy knew how deep the seat bucket and what angle the back wheels should be. She specified fold-up footplates to make it safer getting in and out of the chair. I appreciated her choice of fold-down push hands when I sat next to a wall or when I wanted them unavailable to those "helpful" souls who come along and start pushing your chair without asking.

Eventually my legs had gained enough strength, balance and control that I could walk from the back of my car to the driver seat by holding onto the car roof for balance. Then I no longer disassembled the wheelchair; I just folded down the seat back and it fit in the hatchback, secured with a bungee cord to keep it from rolling around. At 21 pounds, it is an easy lift.

Crutches

It took about two years to transition to crutches, at first using them at

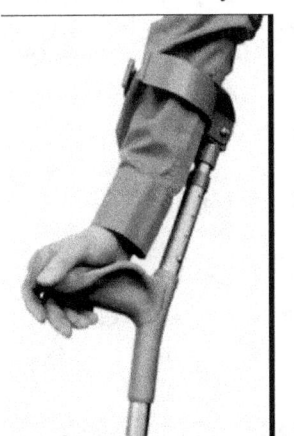

rehab and around the house but still using the walker to go into stores and the gym. Later, I could use the crutches in stores but the shopping cart is also excellent substitute walker. It's possible that people in the grocery store do not think I am disabled, since they are all using grocery carts too. I stand up straight and do my best walking in grocery stores to try to pass as a normal walker for a few minutes.

I used forearm (sometimes called Lofstrand or Canadian) crutches from year 2 to year 5 of my recovery. They balance leg movements, right crutch striking the ground as the left foot takes a step. The motion is closer to walking than pushing a walker. I was able to stand up straighter, fit through narrower openings, see where I was going and walk faster.

I blame my crutches and wheelchairs for most of the damage to my thumbs. My thumbs worked hard during the years I was propelling my own wheelchair. If my legs got tired or spastic when I was on crutches my arms took over and much of my body weight transferred to my hands. The handles on the crutches pressed hard on the joints at the base of my thumb. Those joints are tender all the time now. Despite periodic cortisone injections, they are so tender that they sometimes hurt just getting a manicure or playing piano.

I did find forearm crutches with handgrips that are a little easier on my thumbs, definitely worth it for anyone using crutches for more than a few weeks.

Hand Controls

When I returned home from the hospital, I depended upon Lynn to chauffeur me to doctors, rehab, shows and work. We found the best hand control firm in our area and they recommended a wonderful hand controls driving instructor. Hand controls can only be installed after the driver is certified to use them. Because my hiatus from driving had been only a few months and I did not have 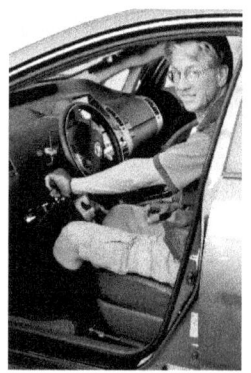 any upper body or brain impairment, I earned my certificate in just one session. Nevertheless, I kept to neighborhood streets for a couple weeks until I was completely confident on my own. Teary-eyed, Lynn watched me drive off, proud of my independent spirit but fearful of the risks.

Hand controls are counter-intuitive. You press the lever forward to stop and down to accelerate, contrary to the joystick moves many of us learned playing video games. Now I make all the moves reflexively and cannot imagine how anyone uses feet to drive a car or why you push the joystick forward to go faster in a video game.

Some patients who have brain injuries or have not been driving for a while take more sessions before they earn a hand control driver certificate. Some rehabilitation clinics offer simulators that make it possible to log practice time before getting behind the wheel of a real car.

The modifications to accommodate quadriplegics are quite amazing. I have seen a quadriplegic friend of mine at the rehabilitation clinic drive his power wheel chair out of the clinic on his own, hit the remote control to open his van with an automatic ramp, drive up the ramp, lock himself into the driver's position, hit the remote again to retract the ramp and close the back door, then drive off using just fingers to steer, accelerate and stop.

My hand controls are much simpler. My arms and head move normally, so I only need modifications for the accelerator and brake. An ingenious lever system attaches to the back of the brake and accelerator so that the car is still drivable in the normal manner by able-bodied drivers. The rods connect to a single lever on the left side (usually) of the steering wheel that directly presses the accelerator down if I pull the lever down and presses the brake down if I push the lever forward.

Gym Strength Machines

Starting at outpatient rehab and later on my own at a commercial

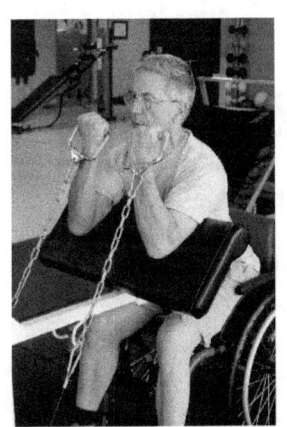

gym, I got back to the "gym rat" life I had enjoyed for decades before the tumor. My upper body recovered to its former levels in a few months. The legs made rapid progress (the good news) but are still a long way from the strength they had before the surgery (the bad news).

The upper body machines include shoulder abductor / adductor, bicep curls, triceps push down, biceps curl, shoulder press, pull up, overhead press, upright row, pectoral flies. Lower body calves, hamstrings, quads and gluts get one or two machines each. I press back against resistance to work my lower back. I hold a two-minute plank for my abs. I balance one foot on a Bosu ball (with my hands on a nearby wall if needed to prevent a fall) to work my lower legs. Then I balance with both feet not holding on with the Bosu ball upside down. These workouts always include stretching. Besides all the strength work I walk in the pool, walk next to the dance barre, walk on the treadmill and/or pedal a recumbent bicycle.

I have shopped gyms to find places where it is least risky to get in and out of the pool, in and out of the showers and easiest to access the particular pieces of equipment I need most. The culture of a gym is often very accommodating for disabled persons, but not always. I have had to deal with club managers who see no need to put signs up to designate a shower for handicapped members only. I have been cursed out for asking a non-disabled member in the only handicap accessible shower how much longer he was going to be showering.

Treadmill, elliptical, bikes and stair machines

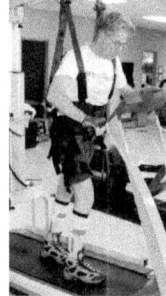
With a harness keeping me upright I started using a treadmill in my first month out of the hospital – and I have been trying to imprint the pattern of faster walking, narrower strides and better form with aerobic machines ever since. After five years, I could walk 15 minutes on a treadmill at over two mph and a two per cent incline. 2.3 mph is the threshold for "normal" walking speed for men of my age. 20 minutes is the threshold for getting some aerobic benefit from the exercise.

After the first year, I could support myself on the machines with my hands and did not need the harness. The elliptical walker has raised-edge footplates which give me more confidence that my feet will not slip off. Stair machines are the hardest challenges for both strength and balance. I can manage only a few minutes, probably not enough to be doing me much good.

Bikes have been difficult. I need straps over the pedals to keep my feet from coming off. Even then, I need to watch my feet most of the time to keep my toes slammed forward under the straps. After five years, I could do a seven-minute one-mile pedal on a recumbent bike. Sometimes the upright bikes make it easier to keep my feet on the pedals, although getting on and off is a little trickier.

E-Stim

One of my PTs suggested an Empi system and my insurance company okayed it. Electric stimulation (e-stim) is recommended for muscle development, pain management and spasticity. The electrodes stick on either end of the muscle to be developed, relieved of pain or calmed from spasm. The unit gives choices for type of pulse, length of time the pulse continues, time between pulses and strength of pulse. I usually choose a pulse that builds up and eases off gradually. For length of time and strength, I usually dial up to a point of discomfort then step back a bit from that. If it is a muscle I cannot feel, then I look at the muscle while it is being zapped and stop increasing the pulse once I see the muscle reacting to the stimulation. I am generous with the space of time between pulses, especially with spastic muscles. If they have a few seconds, spastic muscles have a better chance of relaxing a bit between pulses. It can be uncomfortable and counterproductive to zap a muscle so hard or so frequently that it stays in contraction (spasm) all the time.

When my activity was limited by a broken fibula in 2011, I kept some muscle development going with e-stim. I have not had great success with e-stim managing spasticity or pain. E-stim is risky above the diaphragm as the electric pulses can interfere with your heart.

Bioness
This specially adapted and engineered e-stim system stimulates lower leg muscles to fire at the right point in every stride. It requires some careful fitting and adjusting, including trial and error with the variety of available electrodes sizes and materials. It is often prescribed for one leg, but – after a donnybrook with my insurance company – I got Bioness systems approved for both legs. They helped me overcome some toe dragging that my legs were doing that caused many near falls. My leg would feel like it was taking a normal stride but the toe would not come up and my leg could not swing forward to take the next step. Because I was using forearm crutches most of the time during that stage of my recovery, I was able to catch myself from falling forward, but it was a scary problem that needed to be fixed.

The Bioness system has a small onboard microprocessor about half the size of a cell phone. It takes input from a pressure switch under the wearer's heel to start a sequence of zaps to get the foot to make a normal footfall, roll from heel to toe, push off and lift the toe for the swing forward to the next step. I used the Bioness system for half an hour or so each day for about six months. The left toe still stays down and pitches me forward on occasion, but it is much improved.

A later issue was more with my knees. My right knee bends pretty much as it should, my left knee does not bend enough. To compensate, my left hip raises up and my left leg whips in a semicircle forward. Five years into rehab, my PT tried the Bioness system again without any significant improvement in my gait. Too bad. Now my old brain has to consciously cue each portion of my stride. Sometimes my head is more tired than my legs after walking practice.

Mobility Scooter

This device might be the most reasonably priced of all the disability gadgets. And I acquired it much later in my recovery than I should have. If I had come out of the hospital with a scooter, I could have managed the months when I was still working and also going to rehab much better. The energy I spent propelling my wheelchair

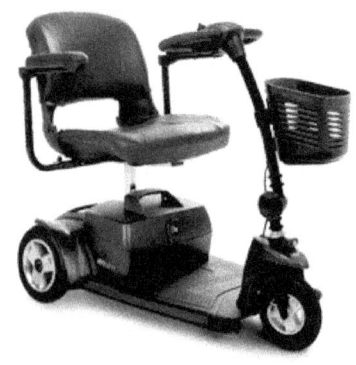

around the school campus could have been greatly reduced.

The insurance issue got in the way. The Ti-Lite wheelchair was so much more expensive than the scooter that the PT clinic recommended waiting until the wheelchair claim was paid before getting a scooter. That was a sensible precaution; but, as it turned out, my insurance paid for both without question.

There are important choices with scooters. The three-wheeled scooter is much more maneuverable. In a house with normal doorways and hallways, it is sometimes the only way to go. The downside is that it tips over much more easily than the four-wheeled scooters.

I only rolled my scooter once. I did not get hurt. I was taking a large trashcan down to the curb. As I maneuvered the trashcan from the curb to the street, I leaned far enough to one side to roll the scooter. After I dusted myself off and got the trashcan where it was supposed to be, I put the scooter back on its wheels and got back on it. Fortunately, our quiet street had no passers by just then.

The second advantage of the scooter I chose is its compliance with airline standards. The scooters with non-liquid batteries are fine with the airlines. When we fly I can ride all the way to the airplane door. The airport gate-checks the scooter and I get to my seat using crutches (or later in my recovery, a cane). At the end of the flight, the ramp crew gets my scooter back up to door of the airplane.

The third important advantage of my scooter is its portability. It breaks down into five pieces, each light enough to lift with one hand. Before I could reliably stand without holding onto something solid with one hand, I would drive the scooter to the back of the Prius, take it apart and load the parts into the hatchback with one hand while using the car's bumper to hold my balance with my free hand. It is about a four-minute process. I do my Christmas shopping in large crowded malls on my own.

Stepper

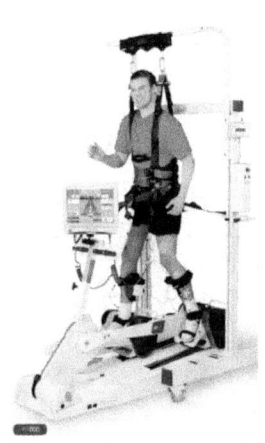

Restorative Technologies makes a whole line of bikes and similar exercise devices that use electrodes to reprogram damaged nerves. The FES bike described above is their product. They also have a stepper that allows the patient to walk with electrodes on the upper and lower legs stimulating each muscle at the right moment for walking. Again, the patient can move on his/her own as much as possible with the machine programmed to zap muscles only as needed.

I was excited to discover this machine and waited a year before one was installed in a location close enough to try out. I was imagining the silver bullet solution: just get on the machine and keep walking until the nerves and muscles were reprogrammed. Alas, no. When I tried it out, the gait the machine produced for me was like stepping off a curb. Heels back, no roll over the toe, no hip coming forward over my toe, butt sticking too far out. A great machine for many paraplegics, but not me.

Nevertheless, I keep watching the announcements and going to the Abilities Expo shows to see if some other company brings out something that fits my needs better.

Trekking Poles

I first saw trekking poles back in my hiking days. They look like ski poles. I walked some of the Appalachian Trail (AT) in Maine, Vermont, New York and New Jersey as well its entire length through New Hampshire. It is so popular that vacationing Europeans often turn up on the trail, many using trekking poles.

I occasionally see patients at PT clinics with trekking poles helping them stand up straighter and keep their eyes up. Therapists working with me would mention them to me, but I did not get a firm recommendation to use them until 2015. By then my thumbs hurt so much using the cane and crutches, that I welcomed any device that takes the pressure off my thumbs. I grip the poles with my fingers and intentionally do not wrap my thumb around the handles. My fingers sometimes get tired and need a rest, but my thumbs get a holiday. With my hands so high, I cannot make my arms and shoulders carry the weight of my body the way they sometimes do with my cane, crutches, Dashaway and walker. So I feel a little less secure, but by 2016 I was using trekking poles at rehabilitation as well as in and out of stores. I could walk a 0.7 mile path in 23:45 or 1.75 mph by April 2016 using trekking poles. The cane still has the advantage of leaving me a hand free to carry things in and out of the store, doctor's office, Starbucks or wherever else I go.

Lights

As I described in the History Chapter, balance depends upon three 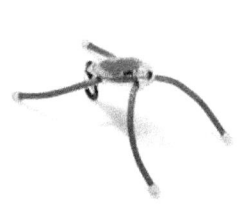 systems: inner ear, sensory and vision. My inner ear is trying to recover and my sensory nerves are mostly gone, so my vision is primarily what gives me what little balance I have left. This was made frighteningly clear when I performed in Twelve Angry Men at the Attic Theater in 2012. I was barely walking on crutches at that point; my shoulders were mostly carrying my weight and my legs would swing forward in what vaguely resembled walking. When we got to dress rehearsal, there were no longer any lights backstage. As soon as I exited the brightly lit stage into the backstage darkness, I suddenly could not tell whether I was horizontal or vertical. My crutches were no help and I grabbed a piece of scenery to reorient myself with some reliable sensory balance.

Gary, an actor friend and an inventor, saw my distress and showed up at the next rehearsal with small flashlights to tape onto my crutches. Perfect. We were excited by Gary's invention and imagined a new business until we did some web searching and discovered we were not the first ones to put lights on crutches or canes. With some further research, I switched to BugLit lights. They are small, very bright and have flexible legs I can wrap around my canes and crutches to keep the light exactly where I want it. They require expensive batteries, however.

Summary

Few devices will help indefinitely. Five years into my recovery my Ti-Lite wheelchair was stored in the garage, along with my AFOs, crutches and my walker. The Empi general purpose e-stim unit and specialized Bioness e-stim units get tried again by PTs every year or so, but without finding any new use for them. The scooter was used less in year five, but still useful for shopping malls, airports and other large venues. My cane with the lights attached and trekking poles were getting daily use.

Notes

The FES bike I rode and the stepper I tried out were supplied by Restorative Technologies. At their website (http://www.restorative-therapies.com/) their entire line of products is described and pictured. Some are even demonstrated on videos.
The bike I used for several months is demonstrated on YouTube at https://www.youtube.com/watch?v=twEsvOldTfk&list=PLuKu1jxc1 6Q57WQlaYat5rA3yoFJyAe8h
The stepper I tried out is demonstrated on YouTube at https://www.youtube.com/watch?v=xEYxSLTBo8Q&list=PLuKu1j xc16Q7s6Gk_-fra_v7CugvO7cpn

Devices: *How a succession of devices advanced my rehabilitation*

Empi TENS units are sold by Amazon and various medical device outlets. I did no comparison shopping. There are lots of all purpose e-stim systems on the market.

Bioness. A number of devices have been developed by this company to make specific applications of electric stimulation to common disabilities caused by stroke, brain injury or spinal cord injury. Their products are unique and can be very helpful depending on the particular patient's needs. In my case, their field support lacked continuity, a different person came out to adjust my devices every time. Their business office was not my favorite. Their web-site is http://www.bioness.com/Home.php

Pride Mobility. This is a great company. They have a wide range of mobility scooters and all the accessories one might need to carry the scooter on a bumper hitch behind the car, with a cargo basket or whatever. http://www.pridemobility.com/

Dashaway. Another great company and a charming inventor, sadly now deceased. Dashaway.com.

Ti-Lite. These made in America wheelchairs are custom fit to the body dimensions of the user. I got mine in red (I am a Red Sox fan) and with front wheels that light up as they turn. I was just being whimsical when I asked for the lighted wheels, but they turn out to be a great safety feature. When we are out at night, the lighted front wheels make it easier to see me crossing the parking lot in the wheel chair. Tilite.com

Various ergonomic forearm crutches are available. It is worth the trouble to try out the options before buying. Start with a web search on "ergonomic forearm crutches".

My car's hand controls were installed by Aeromobility. http://www.aeromobility.com/. Their expertise made the hand controls on our cars much easier to use than the ones we have met in rental cars.. Aeromobility also has a full range of wheelchair-accessible cars and vans. It's a family-owned company with wonderful customer service and professionalism.

Devices: *How a succession of devices advanced my rehabilitation*

Abilities Expo shows have convention-like events in major cities around the country. You will see all the products and services for people with disabilities on a large venue floor where you can actually demo some of the devices. Abilities.com.

I get the BugLit miniature flashlights I use on my canes and crutches for night time visibility at Amazon. I get the batteries there as well.

Remember, all of the internet sites in this book can be reached through http://tinyurl.com/StacyHolmesAuthor. You will not have to type in each site I like in the book. Go to this one site and you can easily click on any site mentioned in this book.

FISH! Philosophy
How playful team-building helps recovery

Around 2001, while I was wrapping up my time as District Superintendent of the Southern Westchester (NY) Board of Cooperative Educational Services (BOCES), one of the trainers brought the FISH! Philosophy video to my office. Jim wanted my approval to offer FISH! Philosophy seminars to schools in our area. We screened the 15-minute video in my office and I immediately approved it as a new BOCES offering.

I had been a superintendent for half my then 30 years in public education when I saw the Fish video. My career was a success story, becoming a principal at 24 and superintendent at 35. But at that moment the job was no fun. I was avoiding people, haunted by distractions and emotionally in the dumps. I did not trust the board of education that hired me, nor some of the senior staff that I had to rely upon to lead a service agency of more than 1200 employees. Just the moment to learn the FISH! Philosophy.

The FISH! Philosophy is most often encountered in a short film that many organizations use for employee team-building and motivation. In the early 1990s, the manager of Seattle's Pike Place Fish Market came up with some ideas to make the repetitive, messy, heavy and intense work of his fish market better for his employees and customers. It worked. For decades to come, Pike Place Fish Market became an entertaining stop for tourists and a workplace emulated by organizations worldwide. As well as a great place to buy fish. There are four pillars of the philosophy:
- Play – make your work fun.
- Make Their Day – include customers and co-workers in the fun.
- Be There – be present in the moment.
- Choose Your Attitude – go through the day with the attitude that *you* choose, not a reaction to others or circumstances.

After that pivotal moment when Jim showed me the video, I would buy stuffed animal fishes and toss them out in staff meetings to recognize individuals who had done something that exemplified one of those pillars. Some teachers took similar approaches with their students and even their own families. I introduced myself to my staff in my next three jobs using the FISH! Philosophy and approached my work with those four pillars very much in mind. Perhaps most important, the bosses, colleagues and clients I sometimes allowed to affect my attitude no longer had that power in my life. As much as possible, I chose my own attitude – no matter what happened at work or anywhere else.

Satisfaction surveys became popular in the latter years of my career. Parent satisfaction and employee satisfaction improved in all three of these administrative posts from one year to the next in my administration. Fewer employees chose to leave my schools and applications for work in my schools increased. Attendance rates, achievement in state testing programs and other student measures all improved. I give the Fish! Philosophy most of the credit for my success in these last three positions. They were not my loftiest or biggest jobs, but my favorites by far.

When I emerged from surgery at Cedars-Sinai Medical Center unable to walk or even roll over in bed, I was back to my pre-FISH! Philosophy days. Life was not fun for me or for anyone working with me. I was so distracted I was hardly present in the immediate moments of daily life. When I wasn't utterly depressed, I was emotionally combative.

In another week, on a rehab unit in that same hospital, I began to remember some of the Fish concepts that made the last 10 years of my career the best:

Play
Play at rehab became competitions with myself. From those early days to now, I count how many times I can repeat a strength-building exercise and remember the number to motivate the next game I play with my body tomorrow.

Mixed into my new life's straining against my limits are other activities that are easy for me. Instead of play in the competitive sense, I just have fun. I'm riding my mobility scooter window shopping at the mall, driving my hand-controlled car to take our granddaughter to gymnastics or playing computer games. My wife attributes our long and joyful marriage in part to my only playing bridge against a computer all these years, never with her.

Make Their Day

Make Their Day started at the hospital rehab unit thanks to great relationships with the occupational therapists, physical therapists, psychologist, recreational therapists, aides, nurses, and doctors. I tried to make the sessions they had with me fun for them. This was a stark turnaround from the early days after the surgery when I was far from anyone's favorite patient.

In the rehab unit, I was happy to see the staff, interested in their careers, ready to chat about current events (I watched a lot of news programs in the hospital) and quick to laugh at my clumsiness. More than five years later, I strive to be one of my physical therapist's, massage therapist's, doctor's and even fitness gym's favorite customers.

My rehabilitation is powerfully motivated by my desire to make my wife Lynn's day. I can manage to get the trash barrels down to the curb each week, shop for groceries, do laundry and clean up the dinner dishes. Helping out makes my day as much as it makes hers.

Be There

For workers, being present in the moment means dismissing all distractions and focusing entirely on the customer, co-worker or student there with you at the moment. A disabled person needs

> Nothing is worth more than this day.
> Goethe

to be even more intensely present. If I am not completely concentrating in rehabilitation, I cannot get myself from sitting to standing. So many physical acts that used to be automatic or simple reflexes require intense focus now. If I am walking on my cane and happen to remember something I need to do, the next moment I may be catching myself from a stumble because I was not keeping complete attention on my walking.

Being present in the moment is important to me for the long term as well. I do not spend much time reliving events in my recovery or further back in my life thinking that I could have made a better choice. Nor do I obsess over whether I will ever be able to get through an airport without using a mobility scooter, walk my daughter down the aisle at her wedding or perform on stage without crutches. I stay present in today's therapy session, gym workout or daily activities. Rehashing yesterday or rehearsing tomorrow diminishes today.

Choose Your Attitude

Choose Your Attitude has always been the most important pillar of the FISH! Philosophy to me. My career changed when I started choosing my attitude toward work, rather than allowing a conniving board member, passive/aggressive boss or philandering employee to make me angry or depressed.

Whether at work or later as a rehabilitating paraplegic, a better attitude was available just by dismissing the unwanted attitude. I identified my anger, frustration, sense of betrayal or depression as originating with someone or something else, not me. I asserted myself, seized control over my attitude and told all the antagonists to stay off my attitude. At work, it helped to change my focus from the meeting, the self-promoting liar or the boss gushing over the latest fad in education. I could reclaim my attitude by hanging out with the students on the playground, the parents dropping off and picking up their children, or with the teachers wrapping up another hectic day late in the afternoon.

Sometimes it is harder to adopt the attitude you want. Depression, anger, sorrow and many other mental health monstrosities are hard to defeat. Spending my life in education may have made it easier for me to accept that you can *learn* to be happy. It turns out you really can go to a lecture, study a book and learn to be happy. For help finding the attitude you want for yourself, I recommend Tal Ben-Shahar. His course at Harvard University was the most popular of all the undergraduate courses at the school for many years. His book Happier reports many ways people find happiness across many cultures. A one-hour overview of his research is available in a wonderful YouTube video. The link is in the Notes at the end of this chapter.

Since the tumor, I have been blessed with mostly excellent medical and therapeutic care. But I have learned to approach every session – good or bad – as a chance to learn and improve, whether because of or in spite of the person working with me. I need to "choose an attitude" that will "make their day", after all.

I see my pain in the alternative; better to hurt than to have nerves so damaged that I feel nothing. I greet each day as my one chance to get better or get worse, dismissing the fantasy that my 67-year-old disabled body will somehow stay stable if I don't keep working it. I wisecrack to relieve dull conversations, enjoy friends/ fellow patients/ family and laugh at mindless drivers on the highway.

Summary
This is but one of the perspectives on life that have helped me continue and even enjoy recovering from crippling surgery and a spinal cord tumor. Since FISH! Philosophy was so much a part of my prior life, it made recovery seem more like just another new job rather than a completely different life.

Notes
The FISH! Philosophy video is closely guarded. You have to buy it or find an organization or library that owns it. Here is the trailer: https://www.youtube.com/watch?v=9cHj6Wj0pko

The organization's web site is Fishphilosophy.com. Some of the books about FISH! Philosophy include FISH!, FISH! Tales, FISH! Sticks and FISH! for Life.

Tal Ben-Shahar gives a lot of his thoughts at Happiness in this wonderful one hour video: https://www.youtube.com/watch?v=5-RVECUWOGQ&list=PLW1E_pXbUMuVfG2WEcDu11Fmy_BelQkBf

Fish Philosophy! *How playful team-building helps recovery*

Happier by Tal Ben-Shahar. It is available in hardcover, electronic and audible formats.

Remember, all of the internet sites in this book can be reached through http://tinyurl.com/StacyHolmesAuthor. You will not have to type in each site I like in the book. Go to this one site and you can easily click on any site mentioned in this book.

Relaxation
How "down time" keeps body and mind going

I have persisted with rehabilitation pretty much non-stop for more than five years – pushing atrophied muscles and disconnected nerves to do some of what they used to do before the tumor. My independence and mobility have surpassed expectations because I have kept at my program. Not everyone faces challenges like mine, but everyone does have some program to keep doing. Diet, exercise, addiction recovery, training, care giving, a job, therapy or rehabilitation – count yourself lucky if you only have one or two of these to manage every day. Whatever it is, it often is not easy physically or mentally to keep at it for five years or five months or even five weeks. Yet, if it is worth doing at all, you really ought to keep at it for the rest of your life.

It has not always been easy for me to get to the gym or rehab or even do my stretches one more time before getting in bed at night. But I stayed with the program, partly because the program had breaks in it. Some breaks were planned, some were unavoidable exhaustion, and some were spur of the moment. I could sense my body and/or my mind was at its limit. When I got that sense, I learned to take a break.

Early in my recovery I was not so smart. Frustrated with my disabilities, I would keep pushing. I told the PT in the hospital during one session that I wanted to keep going with the walker. He told me my feet were not moving anymore; my legs were worn out. My mind was pushing even when the muscles were so tired that they could not move my foot another inch.

> Each day should have a clearly marked emergency exit sign.
> Dr. Sun Wolf

Pushing workouts too far extends my recovery time afterwards exponentially. A day to recover from a big workout becomes three or more days of spasms and cramps after too big of a workout. Mental exhaustion becomes depression.

Relaxation: *How "down time" keeps body and mind going*

This chapter is about some of the ways I gave my mind and body relaxation that made the exertion just completed feel worthwhile and the upcoming workout welcome.

Meditation

Most of my life I would have been chosen as the person in the room least likely to meditate whether I was at work, a neighborhood gathering, among family or anywhere else. Intellectual, self-absorbed and ambitious, I drove my life hard from one cup of coffee to the next. Even my play had competitive goals, miles to cover on the hiking trail, games to win on the computer or rabidly following the Red Sox (and knowing exactly what they should have done when they did not win).

My first encounter with meditation was at a summer institute for public school superintendents held at Harvard University. Each day of the week long institute featured two or more sessions with experts from fields other than education. This was, after all, down time for harried school leaders; we were eager to hear about anything *except* public education for that one glorious week away from the grind.

One professor, whose name I cannot remember, was from Harvard Medical School. A highly regarded cardiologist, he was a long way from an eastern mystic wandering in from the desert after a month of ascetic contemplation. Like me, he was someone you would never expect to meditate. He advocates meditation, he said, only because it makes his patients live longer. He had two groups of patients with heart trouble, those that meditated and those that did not. Those that meditated did not have as many or as frequent or as serious recurrences of their cardiac problems. This same physician/ professor somehow found his way into one of Boston's more troubled schools. He found students who were stressed by their lives in poverty, the physical danger of their neighborhoods as well as their struggle to succeed at school. Some of these students were willing to meditate a few minutes each school day. Their attendance, behavior at school and academic performance exceeded those of students who did not meditate.

Relaxation: *How "down time" keeps body and mind going*

I was even more impressed when I experienced what a simple process this cardiologist/ researcher was calling "meditation". He asked us all to relax while still in our chairs, close our eyes and pay attention only to our breathing. We were not to count the breaths, repeat any syllables, hold any pose or move. When some thought would come into our minds, we were to simply let it go and continue paying attention only to our breathing. Even in what was just a demonstration of his methods, many of us felt we had a pleasant break while meditating in that simple way. If that was all one needed to do to live longer or do better in school, what a great discovery!

In the years to come I remembered that experience from time to time and would meditate to clear my mind and have an interval of peace in times of great stress. I never studied with a meditation guru or even read a book. I just stopped, relaxed my body as best I could, paid attention only to my breathing and dismissed any thoughts that came into my mind, inwardly saying "Oh well..." as I let them go.

In the hospital, I meditated to pass the time between when my physical therapist or occupational therapist was supposed to arrive and when s/he actually showed up. I found myself getting all wound up by their chronic lateness, imagining how much longer it would take me to recover because of my diminished time in PT and OT sessions. So I started meditating a minute or two before the appointment time and continued until the therapist arrived. Whether the session started on time or not, I was peacefully ready for it.

Then there are the MRI sessions. MRIs are very noisy, the radiologists are looking for more bad stuff inside my body, and they will not tell me the results for at least two days. Scary thoughts in an intimidating environment. I focus on my breathing instead. I do the same during radiation treatments. The claustrophobia of the restraints and the anxiety over whether the radiation gun is aimed at the right place are the first things to put out of my mind as I pay attention, again in a very noisy place, only to my breathing.

Relaxation: *How "down time" keeps body and mind going*

Massage

As our careers have taken us to another of the ten homes in six states where Lynn and I have lived, we have sought out massage therapists for occasional or regular therapy.

Once settled in California, I met Ernie at one of the shops in a regional chain of spas near our home in Mission Viejo. He has since gone out on his own and brings his portable massage table to our home twice a month. A Marine veteran with experience in the Wounded Warrior project, he is not a soothing, gentle masseur. Mine is not the first busted up body he has had on his table. He worked on me a few times before the surgery, so he and my family doctor are the only professionals who have seen the whole progression from my prior condition, through my disability and thus far into my recovery.

Massage therapy allows me to give my body to Ernie for 90 minutes. I do not have to make anything move or wonder where my foot is. He lifts, pulls, stretches, kneads and moves me. I get to be totally passive. Ernie's memory amazes me. I am just one of many disabled persons he treats (he has some world class athletes as clients as well), but still he remembers what response he has gotten from various parts of my body going back for years. I was so encouraged when he pressed hard on the middle of my right foot, for example, and asked me if I could feel it. "I feel pressure on the bottom of my right foot," I answered. He went on to tell me he had pressed that same point months earlier with no response, then an involuntary jerk for a couple months until that day when I could consciously feel his pressure. No one has mapped the creeping recovery of deep tissue and even light touch sensation in my lower body better than Ernie. His work is definitive proof every other week that my nerves are still waking up. Albeit very slowly and very gradually.

Mani / Pedi

A triumph – transferring from my wheelchair to the fancy recliner where you can sink your feet into a whirlpool bath before the pedicure. Some anxious owners and stylists looked on but I got the edge of my butt onto the chair then used my arms to pull my body along. My right foot does not feel hot or cold, so I learned to put my left foot in first to test the water temperature. My left foot recovered light touch sensation in stages. For a few months, the filing of my toenails was reported over my damaged nerves as pain. I was happy to be feeling anything. A year later, trimming and filing my left toenails felt normal, not unpleasant at all. The right foot toes tingle and sometimes jerk a little, but they still do not send any messages that make it all the way back to my brain. The scratchy brush scrubbing the bottoms of my feet wakes up a few nerves, again more on the left than the right.

The simple pleasure of the nail salon is one more normal thing I can still do independently. Relaxing in the chair with the cushions providing mechanical massage is precious down time for me, a break after a hard workout at the gym or a welcome respite after running errands.

Scooter Time at the Mall

Beyond a few trips during Christmas season, I probably do not go to the mall five times in a year, but most of those are very therapeutic. I sometimes feel myself hemmed in by how hard it is to move around a store, even using a shopping cart as a walker. Or I get cranky over how much attention it takes to just keep my balance as opposed to actually looking at the merchandise and how impossible it is for me to stroll through more than one store without becoming exhausted.

My scooter comes to the rescue. Without needing anything, I grab a handicap parking spot right next to the walkway from the parking garage to the Shops at Mission Viejo Mall. I spend an hour or two getting around the mall faster and easier than anyone else there. I might buy a latte at Nordstrom's café and/or a Bailey's Shake at Hagen Daz (or both), but the rest of it is just cruising, people watching and getting around a large shopping mall almost effortlessly.

Psychologically it feels like a reward for all the hard work that got me to the point of exhaustion and frustration. No more fighting with a wheelchair, walker, crutches or whatever; I just enjoy a break riding the scooter.

Relaxation: *How "down time" keeps body and mind going*

Road Trips

We break the routine on a bigger scale with 3 to 6 road trips each year. We have ventured up to Sacramento when daughter Emily's veterinary practice and her fiancé Steven's college studies were centered in Sacramento and UC Davis. Lynn's brother Jim lives near San Francisco with his wife Dana and daughter Kit. His grown sons are in San Jose and San Luis Obispo. Sometimes we make stops to see the whole family. Jim has his own advertising company.

We have also driven to Tucson to visit sister-in-law Merrilee, her sister Gail and Gail's husband Ed. We take in theater performances, spring training baseball, book festivals at the University of Arizona, some great restaurants and the area's many parks.

California seems to have wineries just about everywhere. We have enjoyed do-it-yourself wine tours in Napa Valley, Santa Ynez and Temecula. I still know almost nothing about wine, but Lynn has become something of a connoisseur. We relish these days, because there is no schedule. We might hit four or five vineyards in a day; but visiting only one or two is just as much fun if we happen to find a nice spot for a leisurely lunch or some fun shopping. Mixing jaunts on my cane at some vineyards with easier rides on my scooter at others means I can get exercise but still have enough energy to enjoy a full day of fun.

Thanks to grandchildren Kyle, Amanda and Emma, we have day-tripped to many athletic events for karate, tae kwon do, gymnastics, roller skating, football and track. Some of the regional and state competitions have turned into overnight road trips. We enjoyed eight-year-old Emma's wide-eyed enjoyment of her first stay in a big city downtown hotel when she competed at the state level in gymnastics at the San Diego Convention Center. We traded points to stay in the flagship Marriott right next door.

Road trips combine a break from routine PT and gym sessions with adventurous ways to keep my activity going using hotel fitness centers and nearby gyms. In many ways our life "on the road" is similar to our time at home, but it still feels like a relaxing break from the ordinary along with the fun of discovering good places to workout, eat, explore, shop and play. Before the driving and adventuring gets tiresome, we are back home feeling refreshed and eager to settle back into our lives at home.

Movie Nights

We have about forty TV shows programmed into our video recording system, so we have entertainment waiting for us most evenings. Fast forwarding through commercials, we watch half-hour programs in twenty minutes and hour programs in forty minutes. We multi-task while watching these shows. I might sift through email on my laptop; Lynn might check Facebook on her Kindle; both of us enjoy computer games. Before long, we are ready for some dessert and sleep. As enjoyable as this time is at the end of the day, it is part of everyday life – nothing special.

Movie nights break this pattern. With so many movies available on DirectTV, Amazon and Netflix, we have only to shop around through the on-screen directories to find a movie that captures our entire attention. We put aside the multi-tasking and curl up like much younger kids enjoying a night at the movies together. Popcorn sometimes. Wine and cocktails always.

Summary

Whatever form the break might take, stopping the grind of gym and rehab time is essential. I could not have kept at my rehab as consistently as I have without breaks during the day every day and the occasional longer escape that brings a change of scene, reunion with friends / family and or some other non-routine activity.

Relaxation is sometimes a celebration of some physical task I have accomplished, such as getting from a wheel chair into a pedicure lounge chair at a nail salon. Relaxation is always time away from routines that, like any routines in life, can become too familiar. Relaxation provides the time to learn about wines, discover a new movie or keep up with family / friends that may be missing from days when energy, time and focus are committed to recovery. These changes of pace always set me up to get back to rehab with refreshed enthusiasm.

Relaxation: *How "down time" keeps body and mind going*

Notes

The teachers in my school sent me all kinds of gifts during my inpatient month at Cedars-Sinai Medical Center. Meditation for Dummies was in one gift basket. I found it a simple unpretentious introduction to meditation. There is nothing wrong with getting into one of the various spiritual belief systems that feature meditation, but it is not necessary.

We have lived in Springfield, Vermont; Oak Bluffs, Massachusetts; Bloomingdale, White Meadow Lakes, Boonton Township and Madison, New Jersey; Ridgefield, Connecticut; Novi, Michigan; Trabuco Canyon and now Mission Viejo, California. We can attest to quality massage therapists in every one of those cities. (There are also contractors good at putting in new kitchens in each place, too.)

Wounded Warrior is a charitable organization to provide services and support to injured military men and women. Woundedwarriorproject.org

Lynn's brother's advertising business: http://www.sanderson-studios.com/index.html

Lynn's nephew Justin's Apple Computer repair business: http://www.mactoschool.com/

Remember, all of the internet sites in this book can be reached through http://tinyurl.com/StacyHolmesAuthor. You will not have to type in each site I like in the book. Go to this one site and you can easily click on any site mentioned in this book.

Good to Great
How to run rehabilitation like a business

Jim Collins is a business consultant, speaker and author with six best sellers focused on American business growth, greatness and sustainability. He researches big profit-making corporations. Later in his career he also ventured into enterprises where greatness is not measured in economic terms (US Marine Corps, public schools, the Girl Scouts and churches, among others), but he has never gone, as far as I know, where I will take his ideas in this chapter: *disability management*.

His biggest seller is Good to Great, published in 2001, with more than 2 million hard-cover books sold. In this book, Collins researches broadly across American business to find what is common among "good" companies that made the leap to "great" ones. He tests his findings by seeing if a great company stays great over time.

Perhaps he is smarter and more insightful than the legions of business students and MBA program professors who conduct the same research. But what I think sets Collins apart from the worldwide oversupply of MBAs is his communication skill. He takes all the technical data that can only be understood by business analysts and scholars then reports it in a way that makes sense to the rest of us. So much so that everyone reading his books or hearing his presentations can take away a personal plan of action when they return to work or, in my case, when I return to managing my rehabilitation.

Before going any further in Collins' teachings, there is an important lesson just in looking at his own personal success. It models for us an important profile for the kind of people we want as doctors, therapists, instructors and care givers. We do not want the doctors treating us to be like most business analysts who could never write a book that millions would understand and value. Doctors who can speak of my condition using medical jargon understood only by other doctors do not help me. Therapists who can accurately describe what is wrong with me, but cannot use their findings to create relevant treatments are no better.

I want my team to include doctors who can use medical jargon to collaborate effectively with all the other medical people, but those doctors also must talk to me and talk to me intelligently. Doctors who condescend to give me an oversimplified "dumbed down" version of their diagnosis or course of treatment are worse than those who do not even try. The greatest shortcoming of highly specialized and elite schools in business and medicine is often the utter inability of their graduates to communicate with anyone except each other.

Collins is an Ivy Leaguer possessing business jargon and advanced analytical expertise that most people could never follow, but he communicates to them anyway. He uses elegant metaphors that represent his recommendations for action without dumbing down his research and findings. His many metaphors gave me powerful ways to approach the many schools and school districts that I improved in my professional life. And now, his school bus metaphor in particular is very much in my mind as I organize the team that helps me get better as a disabled person.

Collins uses the metaphor of the school bus to represent an organization. The person in charge is driving the bus as well as deciding who gets on and who gets off the bus. Taking an organization from good to great involves:

- Getting the right people on the bus
- Getting the wrong people off the bus
- And getting the right people in the right seats on the bus.

Collins' research concludes that good organizations that transform themselves into great ones and then sustain that greatness over time do all of those 3 metaphoric functions consistently and well.

For good rehabilitation to become great rehabilitation and sustain that success over time, the effort should be organized and led in a manner that is in harmony with Collins' school bus concepts.

Good to Great: *How to run rehabilitation like a business*

Getting the Right People on the Bus

I have chosen surgeons based on their experience with similar surgeries:

- A urologist who had done hundreds of TURPs before performing that operation on my prostate gland
- An orthopedic surgeon who had rebuilt the shoulders of dozens of football players and many more couch potatoes before working on my rotator cuff
- For my spinal cord tumor, the top spinal cord neurosurgeon with the most experience doing similar surgeries that we could find.

This concept goes well beyond doctors. I chose a wonderful hand-controlled driving instructor who has been at his business a long time, taking over from his father who had taught hand-controlled driving for his career as well. The company that modified our cars specializes in making vehicles work for disabled drivers and passengers. I can really appreciate how good they are when I use hand controls installed by a rental car company mechanic instead.

In choosing organizations, businesses and medical facilities, culture helps determine who should be on the bus. Lynn chose my outpatient rehabilitation facility by walking into likely clinics and talking to the people working there. She had chosen many corporate partners and clients in her professional life by the same process: walking in, looking around and talking to workers. She saw the equipment I would need, a focus on neurological rehabilitation and a PT who loved where he worked so much that he stayed late, showed Lynn around and answered all her questions.

Sometimes the right person on the bus has the critical equipment I need. We chose wheelchair and scooter companies based on the products they sell. Research, checking with other disabled people and recommendations from PTs pointed toward Ti-Lite wheelchairs and Pride scooters, so we found dealers nearby with strong experience and reputations.

Experience, the right culture, the state of the art products, or sometimes all of these factors helped us decide who would be on the bus.

Getting the Wrong People off the Bus

Lynn and I learned to be cautious with referrals. Many doctors, hospitals, clinics, medical supply stores, etc. have networks, even contractual agreements, obliging them to refer patients to others in the network. We learned to ask why a doctor recommended this or that professional or institution and what others they would not recommend so highly and why. These questions allowed us to discount recommendations for college friends, women or men they used to work with and especially those who were just part of the same network. HMO and PPO networks are often composed of those professionals willing to accept deep discounts on their fees for the privilege of processing their bills through patients' insurance companies without any regard to their expertise, patient satisfaction and experience.

These questions allowed me to upgrade some other recommendations. When my family doctor recommended taking my aching thumbs (too much wheelchair pushing and crutch walking) to the same orthopedist that did the doctor's own carpal tunnel repair, I was sold. When my physical therapist went down the long list of reasons she had for choosing Ti-Lite and objectively contrasted the not so good alternatives from other companies, I knew we were working with the right wheelchair manufacturer.

I accept hand-offs from one doctor/ therapist / whatever to another with great reluctance. Hand-offs free up somebody's busy schedule, fill up somebody else's empty schedule, let someone go on vacation, accommodate a high profile patient who just came in unannounced, and so on. Nowhere on that list of reasons to hand me off is "improve services for Stacy". I have learned to cancel appointments if I do not know in advance that the substitute professional is really up to the task. Hand-offs don't get on the bus unless they are good enough to be more than temporary substitutes.

I have worked with at least 16 different interns, mostly in PT clinics. Because I am a retired educator, it is hard for me to decline to work with an intern who needs hands-on experience to complete his/her education. But more than five years of physical therapy have given me perspectives on good therapy, great therapy and clueless therapy. I would volunteer my time outside my regular sessions to let interns practice whatever skills they are trying to master, but I will not forego my regular rehab with a good or great PT to be the training mannequin for a rookie. That is hard for me to say as an educator, as the father of a veterinarian who has been through her own internship and residency or even as just a good natured patient who does not want the clinic to think I am a cranky old man. Nevertheless, I allow my PT to bring any guests including interns that she wants with her when she gets on the bus, but the intern does not get to come on the bus alone.

    I have to temper my little rant about interns with the acknowledgement that Professor Beth Fisher spent that magical half hour with me only because she came out from the university to check on one of her students – the intern who was working with me at the time.

    Much of my purpose in continuing physical therapy for over five years has been the need for therapists who can guard me and coach me through high-risk moves. For example, going up a flight of steps without looking at my feet and sliding my hand only lightly on the banister requires a PT a step or so below ready to catch me when a spasm, misstep or momentary loss of attention leads to a fall. That exercise is not as productive if I have to do it with a white-knuckled intern clutching a gait belt around my middle. I'm better off trying some stairs at the shopping center on my own and trusting my strong hands and arms to grab something solid fast enough if I lose my balance.

    The second strongest reason for continuing physical therapy is the expert analysis and diagnosis of my walking and other physical activity. I have spent months, maybe years working on important activities but not the most critical issues with my gait, strength and balance only to have someone like Professor Beth Fisher or Dr. Mary Beth Pongetti come along and see in an instant what the critical issues are, redesign my rehab plan and kick my functioning to a higher level. Even these superstars who have treated me only became superstars after being just competent young professionals for their first few years.

How much of a good thing to include in my rehabilitation schedule is another tricky issue. I may benefit from PT, but I benefit from going to the gym on my own as well. The gym has dozens of specialized machines. It also has a pool and a dance barre to practice unassisted walking. I can work out for two or more hours at the gym; PT clinics have one-hour sessions. So the PT clinic stays on the bus, but not every day.

I listen to recommendations, but I make the decision that makes sense and feels best to me. I have moved from zero gym sessions on my own per week to one to two to three and back to two all based on who should be on the bus today. It is a little hard to do PT twice a week and gym twice a week and have days off in between; there are not enough days in the week. So there are back-to-back PT and gym days if necessary; because I know PT and gym both need to be on the bus, and once a week is not enough for either PT or gym.

I have learned to stop the bus and let someone get off once in a while. The clinic may have changed its focus or I may have progressed beyond what the therapist can really do for me. After I baked a batch of cookies and washed the dishes in the clinic's kitchen, my occupational therapist stepped off the bus. I may have cherished their friendship, admired their expertise or esteemed their seniority. But if their treatments were not changing my disability or enhancing my functioning, I let them off the bus.

I have let medical specialists and other professionals off the bus who were focused on their careers, products or status at the expense of my improvement and/or others on the team. It would be nice if someone other than me saw the big picture and could formulate the plan for my ongoing rehabilitation, integrating the implications of all my history to date and all the expert input from those working with me, but there is no such person. Those who diagnose, prescribe or recommend without respecting how much they do not know about me and how much they do not know about all the fields of rehabilitation expertise, products, and services besides their own get off at the next bus stop. It is my rehabilitation, not anyone else's. I have to drive the bus. I wish there were a doctor smart enough to read my chart, work with me a few minutes and formulate what my overall treatment should be. But there is no such doctor.

All the people on the bus have to tell me what they know in a way I will understand, resist puffing up their role to be more than it is, help me integrate what they know with what I and the many others on the bus know, and then play their part on the team in a way that helps me and everyone else on the bus. If they also earn a fee, sell a product or make some other personal gain along the way, terrific. I just need to feel that helping me get better is each team member's primary purpose for being on my bus.

Getting the People in the Right Seats on the Bus

Rehabilitation is a lot like a corporate team effort. I have the capacity and the will to run my own rehabilitation as CEO of Stacy's Rehab. I drive the metaphorical bus, albeit with hand controls. I hope to run a great rehabilitation, not just a good one. Other disabled persons may not have the capacity and/or the will to drive the bus; but somebody must. A rehab without somebody carefully choosing who is on the bus and who should get off it is not going to be great and probably not even very good. A great rehabilitation needs a boss or a bus driver. I discovered some other vital seats on my rehab bus over the first years of my rehabilitation:

Human Resources Director
Finding, supervising, evaluating and communicating with all the doctors, hospitals, therapists, clinics, and others takes a lot of time and energy that might be better spent on doing the rehabilitation activities themselves. Lynn has been my HR Director.

Home Accessibility Designer
Making a home safe and accessible is a specialized skill. The Home Accessibility Designer must understand what the disabled person's needs are today and what they are likely to be next

year. This designer must also know what is available. Beds, toilets, all kinds of furniture and almost everything else in a home have accessible models that must be part of the designer's idea book. Finally, the designer must know how to implement his/her design whether with contractors or do-it-yourself. Lynn has dramatically remodeled all of the eight houses we have lived in; with half a century of interior design projects behind her, she took on accessibility design and now includes it in her repertoire.

Family / Tribe
I have not encountered any great rehabilitation that did not have a support system for the disabled person. Some families come together when disability strikes. Some fall apart. One rehab friend told me his wife of 20 years had moved out: "She married me for better or for worse but not for spinal cord injury." For this guy (and others) friends at rehab, in the neighborhood, church, school or anywhere have to be shown new seats on the bus. They may not become family, but they may be his/her tribe. (More about tribes in the chapter on The Element.) My family came together in response to my disability. And I also found supportive tribes at rehab clinics, the gym and the theater.

CaringBridge readers
During my first five years of rehabilitation I posted nearly 2000 entries in my recovery blog. I have depended upon a small core of regular readers as well as a much larger group of occasional visitors to read and to respond to my posts. The pressure of daily posts for nearly four years (I backed off to weekly posts for years four and five) caused me to reflect on each day's progress, frustrations and possibilities, so that I could share it with my readers. An incorrigible entertainer, I found humor, good news and progress to write about on days I might have otherwise let pass without discovering any of that upbeat encouragement.

Surgeon
My surgeon orders annual MRIs of my spine and speaks with me on the phone at least once a year with the good news that my

tumor is stable and not likely to cause any further trouble. He owns the reality that he left me with a body changed forever and a tumor that I will always worry about. When we chat on the phone, he asks how I am doing and I check in on the progress of his research, his family and surgical practice. Surgeons who care about a patient years after the surgery are rare. Safety, efficiency and expertise in the operating room are more important traits to be sure, but the surgeon you want on the bus for more than a day is one who cares about you for more than a day.

Hospital
Cedars-Sinai Medical Center is dysfunctionally large, and I would not return there unless their amazing facilities and doctors could not be matched elsewhere. Creature comforts were scarce, nursing care ranged from amazing to awful, but every room was a single with state-of-the-art equipment. Disabled persons need confidence in the hospital providing their care at their most vulnerable, terrifying and fragile moments in life. I did not have a choice where I would have my surgery, but if I did I would choose someplace where former patients loved the nursing service.

Rehab doctor
I needed a specialist MD in rehabilitation for longer than just the month at the hospital. Two years later when Dr. Rau closed his practice after signing a sweet deal with Kaiser Permanente, I tried finding another rehab doctor, but ended up using my family doctor. There are not that many medical options for my condition anyway. It has worked out fine. I don't need a rehab specialist physician on the bus anymore.

Rehab and SCI insiders
Whether they are friends who happen to be doctors, therapists letting their hair down or just patients with many years of rehabilitation behind them, insiders who will tell me the stuff doctors and therapists usually do not are welcome on my bus. From them, I have learned:

- Almost nobody walks normally ever again after spinal cord surgery. Statistics showing SCI patients "walking" again include those walking with canes, crutches and walkers.
- Try marijuana; nobody knows whether it will help you or not, what kind you should try or how much you should take. Find out for yourself.
- Almost everyone with spinal cord injury gets osteoporosis; put as much weight on your leg bones as possible for as long as possible everyday, even if you can only stand holding on to a walker or the side of your bed. Without daily stimulation, bones get soft.
- Leg braces may protect your knees for a few months but they mess up the way you walk for years. I am still trying to get the balance from my heels across my whole foot and I stopped wearing leg braces more than three years ago.
- Stretching is great, but you can overdo it; long muscles are weak muscles.
- Pushing yourself in a wheelchair and crutch walking wreck your thumbs. Wear hand and thumb protectors even if you do not think you need them. Get physical therapy for your hands BEFORE they start hurting.
- Muscle relaxer pills relax your brain too; fight back with brain work, puzzles and Lumosity.

Family doctor
Spinal cord injury has brought so many professionals into my life that I need someone to help interpret all the input, help me with referrals and support my experiments with new medications, doses and combinations.

Physical therapist
I need a personal relationship with my doctors. I would never be happy in a large family practice with a different doctor seeing me every time. The same is true of physical therapists. I consider the facilities, location and culture of the PT clinic, but I have to have a PT I can trust and rely upon sitting up front on the bus.

Doctoral programs in physical therapy have more content than master's programs. DPTs who have also earned their postdoctoral specialist certificates in neurology are even more prepared to help me. Those with strength certificates (usually earned concurrently with the doctorate) have still another professional training component that will help them treat me more efficiently.

Besides training and a few years treating spinal cord injury patients, the DPT on my bus must have physical skills that make me feel safe and the DPT her/himself feel confident as we attempt physical moves where I may lose my balance or fall. There are not many rookie or 20-year veteran physical therapists with reflexes and strength sufficient to catch spastic old men falling down stairs or off a balance machine. So the DPT on my bus will be a midcareer neurological, orthopedic and strength specialist who plans to be available regularly for the next few years. S/he has and maintains athletic strength and reflexes.

Hand Controls Installer
There are vast differences between the mechanics who install hand controls really well and those who are just adequate. Having hand controls that are smooth and responsive and that do not fatigue my hands, fingers and arms on long trips makes everyday driving and road trips safer and more enjoyable. I have rented cars with hand controls from various rental agencies. I have been disappointed with Hertz, impressed with Alamo and usually impressed with Enterprise.

Hands Control Teacher
Working with someone who teaches a lot of disabled people to drive provided me the benefit of his experience. His confidence that I would learn to drive with hand controls without much difficulty bolstered my optimism as I learned a new skill.

Gym
I had to let one gym off the bus for their indifference to handicap access. After a sweaty work out for two hours in the gym and 15 minutes in the chemically treated waters of the pool, I need a shower with grab bars, a bench and a hand held showerhead.

Good to Great: *How to run rehabilitation like a business*

Appropriate signs, maintenance and a sensitive attitude among the gym members also make the difference between a safe and risky locker room.

Summary
There are many useful metaphors in Jim Collins' work, each a useful tool for applying the findings of his research. The school bus metaphor has helped me particularly. I have to drive the bus of my rehabilitation. I cannot get anywhere unless I have the right people on the bus, the wrong people off the bus and the right people in the right seats on the bus. With all of that done well and consistently, my bus is on its way not to just a good rehabilitation, but a great rehabilitation.

Notes

1994: Built to Last: Successful Habits of Visionary Companies by James C. Collins and Jerry I. Porras
1995: Beyond Entrepreneurship: Turning Your Business into an Enduring Great Company by James C. Collins and William C. Lazier
2001: Good to Great: Why Some Companies Make the Leap ... And Others Don't by James C. Collins
2005: Good to Great and the Social Sectors by James C. Collins
2009: How the Mighty Fall: And Why Some Companies Never Give In by James C. Collins
2011: Great By Choice by James C. Collins and Morten T. Hansen

This is a five minute video that uses cartooning to illustrate a capsule overview of Jim Collins' *Good to Great* book.
https://www.youtube.com/watch?v=Yk7bzZjOXaM

Dr. John Yu, the neurosurgeon who operated on me and continued to check on me and read my updated MRIs five years later is Vice Chair of Neurosurgical Oncology at Cedars-Sinai Medical Center in Los Angeles.

Good to Great: *How to run rehabilitation like a business*

Aeromobility, an outstanding vehicle installer and modifier for everyone from those who have a little trouble walking to quadriplegic passengers and drivers.
http://www.aeromobility.com/ They also provide great referrals to hand-control driving instructors. Depending on the time a disabled person has been away from driving, whether the disability involves the brain and how much upper body impairment s/he has, driver training may be an hour in a hand-controlled car with an instructor or several weeks using simulators in a specialized clinic.

The Accessible Home: Designing for All Ages and Abilities Paperback – October 23, 2012 by Deborah Pierce

My recovery blog is at
http://www.caringbridge.org/visit/stacyholmes/

A medical research article analyzing which spinal cord injury patients are likely to walk again:
http://www.ncbi.nlm.nih.gov/pmc/articles/PMC3952432/

Keeping your brain sharp is a challenge at my age. It's a bigger challenge after retirement, with muscle relaxer drugs hitting my system three times a day, and with big chunks of every day focused on physical exercise without much cognitive challenge. Fortunately, I enjoy activities that help me keep my wits working. I play bridge, hearts, Sudoku, Spider and FreeCell games on my phone. When my laptop is handy, I get into crosswords from USA Today and the LA Times. I play NY Times puzzles on my phone. And I play Lumosity games. Lumosity has an impressive research base to support its series of games designed to improve its users' flexibility, speed, problem solving, focus and memory. They report progress in each category and in comparison to a huge reference group of users by gender and age range. Lumosity.com.

Good to Great: *How to run rehabilitation like a business*

The American Board of Physical Therapy Specialties confers certificates for Doctors of Physical Therapy (DPTs) in eight specialty areas of physical therapy: Cardiovascular and Pulmonary, Clinical Electrophysiology, Geriatrics, Neurology, Orthopaedics, Pediatrics, Sports, and Women's Health. DPTs licensed to practice with 2000 hours of clinical experience in a specialty area are eligible to take the exam to earn the specialist certification. Normally, a year-long professional development course and extensive individual study is required to prepare for the exam. http://www.abpts.org/home.aspx.

Osteoporosis as an almost inevitable consequence of spinal cord injury is discussed in a research study discussed without too much medical jargon here: http://www.abpts.org/home.aspx.

Remember, all of the internet sites in this book can be reached through http://tinyurl.com/StacyHolmesAuthor. You will not have to type in each site I like in the book. Go to this one site and you can easily click on any site mentioned in this book.

Arts
How enjoying and creating give recovery joy and purpose

For all my Type A driven personality and left brain dominance, I have always enjoyed many kinds of art. I never studied art, so I substitute enthusiasm for talent when I perform, whether as a writer, actor, director or piano student. I have opinions and experience instead of art knowledge or training. The word "dilettante" and the phrase "Jack of all trades, master of none..." sum up my creative life perfectly.

In my school career, I championed arts programs as the budget battles and testing schemes steadily pushed arts out of the curriculum and off the schedule. So many students make it through school only because they find one course that really interests them and perhaps with that course a group of students and a teacher with similar passions. For these students, the only reason to come to school and put up with everything else may be a drawing class, a choir, a drama production, a dance studio, a film class or a jazz band.

> An artist is not a special kind of person. Each person is a special kind of artist.
> Unknown

My sister Nancy and sister-in-law Merrilee suggested writing a CaringBridge blog to me when I was first diagnosed with a spinal cord tumor. What a great suggestion! At first it seemed a mere convenience. Blogging my progress would broadcast information to the many colleagues, family, church friends and neighbors who would otherwise keep me and/or Lynn on the phone for hours repeating the same update over and over. But soon I was looking for funny, absurd and hopeful experiences in each day to pass along in my almost daily postings. Expressing my recovery in writing gave me a chance to create something every day. Any day with a few moments to draw, write, sing, act, dance or play is a better day. And so, any day of recovery with a bit of creative writing is a better day.

The creation – whatever it is – lives on after the day is done making that day special, a cherished memory. A remembered song. A selfie with a grin. A sketch. A video shot with a cell phone. I am so grateful that all those thoughts and events from my first years of recovery were written down. It is hard for me to reread some of those times; but, when I want or need to go back, it is reassuring that they are there.

Enjoying Art

Lynn and I found theaters and concert halls in our first few years in California. We subscribed to the Geffen Playhouse, just off the UCLA campus, for a season. We loved the performances but dreaded the drive. It turns out there is no time of day to conveniently get into or out of Los Angeles without a helicopter. Closer to home, we enjoyed many seasons at Segerstrom Arts Center in Costa Mesa, a much easier drive from our home. Next door to Segerstrom is South Coast Repertory (SCR), with both medium and small stages offering mainstream and more *avant-garde* productions respectively. SCR has consistently been our favorite for its choice of shows and quality of its productions as well for its accommodation of my disabilities.

While I was in the hospital, we gave away our season tickets to friends, spending those nights together instead in my room at Cedars-Sinai Medical Center. Soon after my return home, we cautiously began our return to arts patronage. I manually propelled my wheelchair up and down the ramps to get into theaters and concert halls. Not all venues are handicap friendly. Segerstrom ushers, for example, have directed us to the door closest to our seats, even though that particular door is down a flight a stairs.

I learned to ask about the location of handicap seating when buying tickets. It is often the front row and/or last row of the venue. Depending on the size and configuration of the auditorium, better sight lines and acoustics might be enjoyed nearer the middle of the seating area. Even when I was not yet very good at transferring out of my wheelchair, I bought better seats than the handicap designated ones, wheeled to the better seats and transferred to the theater seat using my strong arms to keep my balance and carry the weight when my legs could not manage the maneuver. I was self-conscious about my spastic legs. Whoever sat next to me appreciated my forewarning, but never seemed to mind my jerks and twitches.

Over the next five years we pared down the number of nights we attended shows and concerts to those we enjoyed the most and those facilities that made more than a minimal effort to accommodate disabled patrons. We see our growing circle of amateur actor and musician friends perform in the many smaller venues in our area, which are often easier for me to navigate. We call these outings "date nights" and often go out to dinner before the performance. My energy and jerking legs are making it through the evening a little better with each passing year. I use a cane, trekking poles, crutches or mobility scooter depending on the distances and terrain. Sometimes the weather dictates how I get into the theater. A cane is not enough for the slippery pavement or gusty winds of the occasional stormy day in SoCal.

We watch most films at home. But we make a few trips to the movies each year, especially for the big special effects and 3D productions. We have discovered Cinepolis, theaters with huge recliner seats and waiters to serve cocktails, snacks, meals and desserts. They have excellent sight lines for their handicap accessible seats and sturdy banisters for adventurous paraplegics like me.

I enjoy staying current with new shows and movies. Knowledge of music and theater is a lifelong passion of mine as well as the foundation for my own performing, writing and directing. I am disabled as Lynn and I make our way to our seats. But when the lights go out and the show begins, I am back in a world I have loved since my first solo with my Mom's band at age five, singing for the soldiers at Fort Bliss in El Paso, Texas. It's a world of possibilities limited only by the extent of my imagination, not by how well I walk.

Making Art

Two years into recovery, I found my way back to the community theater stage at The Attic Theater. Playing Juror #9 in <u>Twelve Angry Men</u>, I was able to get on stage and take my seat at the jury table using forearm crutches. Soon after this production, The Attic asked me to direct <u>Pirates of Penzance</u>. In the following year I acted in <u>You Can't Take It with You</u> and <u>Inherit the Wind</u>. I continued directing at The Attic as well: <u>HMS Pinafore</u>, <u>One Flew over the Cuckoo's Nest</u>, <u>The Mikado</u> and A <u>Funny Thing Happened on the Way to the Forum</u>. The last two were especially enjoyable; Lynn joined both productions as Assistant Director and Costumer. I have also given presentations on character acting at arts festivals for area high school students.

Performing has been tremendous motivation for rehabilitation. I tell the PTs that my goals include walking well for the first few steps I take with a cane, so that the audience will not be distracted by any wobbly first steps when I get up to move about on stage. I have challenged myself to extend the length of time I can direct a rehearsal. Getting on my feet during the rehearsal and walking between the rows (supporting myself with the seatbacks in front of me) avoids the cramping that comes with sitting for a long time.. The cumulative fatigue from three months of rehearsals and performances is still daunting. Lynn and I both collapse in utter exhaustion after the closing night cast party.

Piano

I have played piano off and on since college. Of all the many things my Mom taught, music was foremost, so there were always pianos in the house. Sadly, I never studied music seriously. I took beginner lessons for one or two quarters in college. Thirty years later in Michigan, I studied with Wally, a great guy who played in Detroit nightclubs. He gave lessons in the back of a piano store in Novi, Michigan. He whetted my appetite for regular piano study.

Once settled in California, I began calling piano teachers and asking keyboard players for recommendations. I used Wally as a model. An older teacher who would know some of the music I like and someone who could teach improvisation along with sight reading and technique. Improvising after years of classical training is different from improvising for someone like me. I know music theory in my head, but my fingers do not have the years of playing scales and arpeggios that real pianists have. I finally found Teddy, younger than Wally, but familiar with show music and popular music from my era. She is a veteran of many years playing in clubs improvising from a fake book. Like Wally, she taught in the back of a piano store that was an easy stop on my way home from work. When the store closed, Teddy moved her lessons to her home. Most of her students are children and teens, many of them moving on to juried piano competitions. But she also teaches several adults who play just for fun.

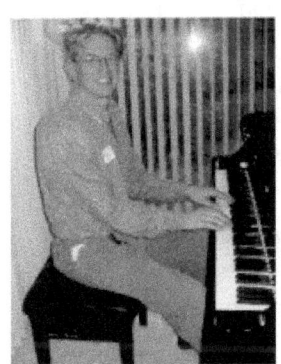

After my tumor had interrupted my weekly piano lessons, I was anxious to get back to them. Starting only a few weeks after the hospital, Lynn would take me to my lessons. I could propel my wheelchair up Teddy's driveway myself, but Lynn would have to tip me backwards in my wheelchair to ease me over the step into Teddy's house. I was back! Within another year, I could drive myself to my lessons with my hand-controlled car and get myself into her house with a walker, then crutches, then just a cane.

My spastic right foot struggled with the piano pedal. I could consciously push the pedal down, but my foot would not stay there if I was not looking at it. So I tied my shoe to the pedal. Over the next years, I gained more control. Still far from normal control and without any sensation of my foot touching the pedal, my pedaling no longer distracts my playing too much. Piano does not require standing or walking, so it has been an accessible creative expression for me from the earliest days of my recovery. Entire piano courses are developed for the adult beginner. Electric pianos that play and feel very much like traditional pianos are much cheaper and much better than they were a few years ago. Beginning or continuing keyboard study is a creative outlet available to many disabled persons.

Writing

Writing about my recovery in a CaringBridge blog has opened a portal to my inner self and exercised my writing so much that now I understand what is going on in my life and what I think about a particular topic only after writing about it. My blogs have included reviews of live shows, concerts, books, TV programs and films. I comment on politics and current events. Connecting to the world through writing overcomes the isolation of retirement and limitation of disability. I have people to talk to in a forum where they are free to join the discussion. The blog allows me to attach YouTube videos and post pictures. I learned the simple process of uploading a video from my phone to YouTube. Once the video is in YouTube, I can attach it to a CaringBridge posting. I can tell the world how it feels to take a step and share the video at the same time.

CaringBridge is free, supported entirely by voluntary donations. Likes and comments from readers are saved along with all the blog entries. I write 99% of the blogs on my site but other sites have multiple authors. There are options for the design of the site. The audience can be completely open, require sign in with email or limit viewing to individuals specifically invited by the author(s). I recommend CaringBridge to anyone in any stage of disability, injury or serious illness. The creative act of writing, choosing pictures / videos to post and designing the site is therapeutic and uplifting. The process keeps friends and family closer and more involved. Recovery is a team effort. Blogging builds and sustains that team.

I have done some writing for the Los Niños de la Calle con Wendy Foundation where Lynn and I both serve. My story recounting my first trip back to see the Red Sox in Boston's Fenway Park appeared in New Mobility magazine. I have supplied testimony, both in person and in writing, to document the need to provide permanent shelter for Orange County's growing homeless population.

Art with Disability Themes

I have a special appreciation for art created or performed by disabled persons as well as art of all sources with disability themes. I am inspired by the strength of others winning their battles to be more mobile, creative and independent, and humbled by the recoveries of those facing handicaps far greater than mine. Perhaps most important, I realize that I am not alone. Others with spinal cord injuries or other disabilities are continuing to recover, many against much greater odds and with much less support than me.

There are many more of us out there sharing through all forms of art than I ever imagined. Here are just a few of my favorites:

Youtube:
- A dancer with only one arm performs with a ballet dancer with only one leg.
  https://www.youtube.com/watch?v=UTrb6i7gJAk
- A mountain bicycle rider in a wheelchair returns to mountain biking, this time on a four-wheeled bicycle.
  https://www.youtube.com/watch?v=WydF4qRwt5c
- My own video kayaking off the Maine coast with son Graham.
  https://www.youtube.com/watch?v=O1zHUP4q5mw
- A motorcycle rider gets back to his sport even after spinal cord injury.
  https://www.youtube.com/watch?v=PddcicrpyZg

Movies
- The Sessions. A man living in an iron lung has sessions with a sex therapist. Sundance Film Festival Award Winner. Trailer:
  https://www.youtube.com/watch?v=Fy2y7UIpgP4
- The Intouchables. A wealthy Parisian quadriplegic chooses as his personal assistant a street-wise young man trying to escape his poverty and rough life. Based on a true story. Another award winner. Trailer:
  https://www.youtube.com/watch?v=34WIbmXkewU
- Forrest Gump. A boy (Gump) with physical and mental disabilities becomes an athletic hero, a war hero, a successful businessman and a husband. Gump (Tom

Hanks) rescues his commanding officer in a Vietnam battle and helps him rebuild his life after his wounds leave him crippled and depressed. A huge critical and box office success as a film, it is also a good book. https://www.youtube.com/watch?v=uPIEn0M8su0

Books
- A Great Deliverance by Elizabeth George. This is the first in a long series of Inspector Lynley Mysteries. The protagonist's close friend and CSI-style crime lab expert is a quadriplegic. They are a team through the entire series of mysteries.
- The Curious Incident of the Dog in the Night-Time by Mark Haddon. This amazing book unravels the killing of a neighbor's dog, family secrets and coming of age from the point of view and in the language of the autistic young boy accused of the crime. There is also a very powerful stage adaption of this work and film as well. Trailer: https://www.youtube.com/watch?v=O704ld5WQnk
- A Whole New Life: An Illness and a Healing by Reynolds Price. An older man stricken by a tumor in his spinal cord (sound familiar?) tells his story of recovery. Price is a poet and author telling his own story. You will not find more beautiful and authentic writing.

Plays, Operas and Musicals
- The Elephant Man by Bernard Pomerance. Based on the life of John Merrick, a horribly disfigured young man who appeared as a sideshow freak was later educated and successfully taken into nineteenth century London society. John Hurt starred in a stage and film version of the story. Trailer: https://www.youtube.com/watch?v=ZvJuJKOmZAY
- Porgy and Bess by George and Ira Gershwin. Porgy is a paraplegic beggar who wins and keeps the love of the beautiful Bess. America's greatest opera is based on the novel by DuBose Heyward who himself was a childhood polio victim and later an invalid with typhoid and

pleurisy. The 75th anniversary film production of opera trailer:
https://www.youtube.com/watch?v=c4rCDMeJIpw

- Richard III by Shakespeare. One of the earliest depictions of a disabled protagonist (albeit an anti-hero) with a complex three-dimensional personage. Laurence Olivier gives the performance other great actors emulate:
https://www.youtube.com/watch?v=5-P0xHwjxiI
- The Curious Savage by John Patrick. Set in a sanatorium a group of mental patients help their new friend in the hospital deal with her difficult family. A community theater promo video:
https://www.youtube.com/watch?v=M0HegJIqQk4
- Cyrano by Anthony Burgess and Michael Lewis. Edmond Rostand's 1897 classic play by the same name is the source material for this brilliant but sadly short-lived Broadway musical where a disfigured artist woos his beloved Roxanne by proxy as he coaches the handsome young man who is in love with Roxanne.

Music
- "The Climb" There is always one more mountain to climb – the anthem for long-term recovery.
https://www.youtube.com/watch?v=QYjl7e0qnhQ
- "One Brick at a Time" from the musical Barnum. Phineas Barnum started from humble beginnings and built his legendary circus one brick at a time. I remember how many bricks there are in a great building as a metaphor for how many "bricks" there are in a great recovery.
https://www.youtube.com/watch?v=d4x2CTooSlY
- "What I Did for Love" from the musical Chorus Line. A dancer falls in the audition for the Broadway show that will make her career. She responds to her career-ending disability with the lyric, "Kiss today good-bye and point me toward tomorrow."
https://www.youtube.com/watch?v=YLQMxgGW_YA
- "Memory" from the musical Cats. An old, bedraggled (disabled?) cat recalls the days when she was beautiful.

The darker times are a metaphorical night at the end of which she sings, "Look, a new day has begun!" The iconic Betty Buckley sang this to me one magical night at the Winter Garden Theater in New York. The theater was sold out, but all the others were just bystanders to Miss Buckley's moment with me. https://www.youtube.com/watch?v=oPEpt051xyM ("Memory" is about 4 minutes into this clip which also includes her Tony Award acceptance speech.)

- "If Tomorrow Never Comes" A Garth Brooks ballad of a man hoping he has expressed his love, so that it lasts forever for his woman even if he does not survive to see another day with her. https://www.youtube.com/watch?v=Rid5sE93axA

Art

- The Wounded Warrior Project Icon https://www.woundedwarriorproject.org/
- Peter Longstaff was a thalidomide baby born with no arms. He paints with his right foot. http://www.mfpa.uk/the-artists/peter-longstaff/
- Photo of eight-year-old Jennifer Keelan crawling up the steps of the Capitol in Washington on March 12, 1990 as part of the campaign seeking passage of the Americans with Disabilities Act. http://www.historybyzim.com/2013/09/capitol-crawl-americans-with-disabilities-act-of-1990/

Summary

Able-bodied or, more accurately, temporarily able-bodied persons as well as those of us already disabled respond to art individually. Each of us chooses what we wear, which car we admire, what new ad on television seems clever and what performer we like. Some of us pick up a guitar, sing along with music on the car radio, sketch a cartoon while on the phone at work, move with music that has a good beat or make up one-liners to joke with friends. Enjoying or creating art allows us to experience feelings and thoughts that help us grow, make us smile and enrich our lives.

Enjoying art as an able-bodied person for sixty years and as a disabled person ever since, I have found it helps me escape sad or difficult moments in life as well as my own shame or inadequacy. The range of what is possible opens up in the world of art. Inspiration that lifts my spirit and motivates my rehabilitation comes freely from so much of the art in my life.

Notes

CaringBridge is a non-profit corporation that hosts blogs for individuals and families with serious illness or injury for free. It provides a website platform through which the individual and all his/her family and friends can communicate. CaringBridge was founded in 1997. By 2006 it was hosting more than 5,000 sites. By 2013 CaringBridge.org tallied 46 million visits. My blog, started in 2010, is at caringbridge.org/visit/stacyholmes.

Geffen Playhouse: geffenplayhouse.com. You can see teaser clips from their productions by searching on Geffen Playhouse in YouTube.

Attic Community Theater is located at ocact.com. My directing includes A Funny Thing Happened on the Way to Forum. A trailer of the production is at
https://www.youtube.com/watch?v=kIMDfzABQFU#
A clip from my leading role in You Can't Take It with You is at
https://www.youtube.com/watch?v=fkTqeJ7TysQ.

Teddy's Piano Studio. http://teddynewsommusicstudio.com/

A wonderful resource listing movies with disability themes:
https://mubi.com/lists/disability-in-film#read-more
This listing also has YouTube clips next to many of the films listed. Many of these films can be watched in whole or in part by searching for them on YouTube.

An annotated list of books with disabled main characters:
http://www.amazon.com/lm/R2QKVETQTJB65C

An illustrated listing of artists painting and drawing with disabilities: http://www.webdesignerdepot.com/2010/03/the-amazing-art-of-disabled-artists/

Photographs of disabled persons at work, home and play: http://disabilityimages.com/

Remember, all of the internet sites in this book can be reached through http://tinyurl.com/StacyHolmesAuthor. You will not have to type in each site I like in the book. Go to this one site and you can easily click on any site mentioned in this book.

Finding Your Element
How to find your element and tribe

In 2006 Sir Ken Robinson vaulted into notoriety with his speech at TED. TED (technology, entertainment and design) spreads ideas in the form of short powerful talks, each eighteen minutes or less, presented at conferences the non-profit organization sponsors. Since 1984, the topics have spread to almost everything imaginable and reached around the world in more than 100 languages. By 2015 TED had made 1900 talks available on their website. TED talks have been viewed over a billion times.

The most viewed of all the presentations over all those years is Ken Robinson's first presentation at TED in 2006. In that speech he told the story of Gillian Lynne, a British school girl whose teachers told her mother to take her to a specialist, certain that she had a learning disorder. Gillian could not complete her schoolwork or keep herself from fidgeting. 80 years later, the description of her 1930s childhood might prompt a diagnosis of attention deficit hyperactivity disorder (ADHD). Today she might be medicated and trained to channel her fidgets with a squeeze toy. Fortunately, her mother consulted a specialist who suggested enrolling her in a dance academy instead of a traditional school. She went on to choreograph blockbuster theatrical hits including Cats and Phantom of the Opera.

Robinson finds almost no opportunity to develop creativity in today's education systems. It is creativity that today's students will need in the future world we educators cannot even imagine today. Robinson asserts that British and American schools have their priorities exactly upside down.

He believes that each person must find his/her element to be happy in life and productive in society. Robinson defines "element" as that thing that you do well and that you love to do. With the curriculum of schools narrowing as a result of undue focus on passing state tests that assess only core academics, it becomes ever less likely that very many students will discover their elements at school.

Finding Your Element: *How to find your element and tribe*

Besides one's element, Robinson writes that each of us must discover her/his tribe to be happy in life and productive in society. One's tribe is composed of like-minded people whose passion in life – their element – is the same as or similar to one's own. For Gillian Lynne, she was much more at home in a dance studio filled with other young dancers even though they were all strangers to her than with neighborhood friends at a traditional elementary school. Again, Robinson criticizes most American and British public schools for narrowing programs to such an extent that there are few tribes one can find in school. One can validate his work by noting the power of the few tribes that do exist in schools, e.g. athletic teams, clubs, gangs and social cliques. Many students pretty much hate school but still attend to be with their respective tribes.

Before my spinal cord tumor, my element was public education leadership. I was good at leading schools and school districts. And I loved doing it. I found my tribe when gathered with fellow superintendents or principals. At the end of my career I was most at home at my own school with my students, their families, my teachers and staff. I was also among my tribe at the gym, where I would stop for a workout on the way home from work about three times each week. I did not have a regular workout buddy or take group classes, but I nevertheless looked forward to and enjoyed time spent with the regulars there. Many I recognized and chatted with, but I rarely saw them elsewhere. Community theater was still another tribe. Sometimes I would act or direct with performers from prior shows but this tribe was more often composed of strangers. Nevertheless, we instantly bonded in our common effort to produce some play or musical. When the show closed many of us were bonded for life, keeping up on social media and attending each other's future performances.

Despite the unsuccessful surgery on my tumor, I initially thought I would just carry on enjoying my life in my element. I went back to work after a month in the hospital and another month of outpatient rehab and trips to the hospital for radiation. I could not drive for the first couple months, but soon (thanks to hand controls) I drove off to work on my own in the morning. I enjoyed the students and managed my school quite well from a wheelchair, but only for a few hours at a time. The time and energy I needed for rehabilitation made working impossible. The small amount of activity I could manage each day was needed for rehabilitation with little left over for anything else. After reducing my work to just two or three days per week for a few months, I retired at the end of the school year.

As a retired disabled person I was in a new world. I was working hard at rehabilitation, but to the world and to my own self I was useless. I was needed on my parents' farms from age nine through high school; I worked full time six months out of every year of college and half time for the other six months (Antioch was a work/study college); I was continuously employed (sometimes with additional part-time jobs) for the next forty years. I was always useful to somebody. Less than a year after the surgery and retired, I was just barely able to take care of myself. I was no longer in my element. Leading schools was over.

I started a CaringBridge blog in 2010. In the five years after the surgery, I grew past daily blogging to do some other writing. I published a piece in <u>New Mobility</u> magazine. After a few unsuccessful attempts, I wrote this book. I have three other books in mind after this one. Almost every morning I get out of bed around eight o'clock while Lynn is still sleeping and I write for an hour or so. I have found my post-spinal cord injury element. I love to write and it is something I seem to do well.

I do not yet have the tribe one would expect a writer to join. There are writing workshops, groups, classes and circles. I have friends who write plays, and a wonderful group that follows my blog, but no tribe of fellow writers.

I don't feel lonely without a tribe of fellow writers. After my morning writing time, I am busy four days a week at physical therapy or at the gym. I help Lynn with the taxi service she operates for our three local grandchildren while their parents are at work. I enjoy tribes at the gym, rehab clinic, granddaughter Emma's gymnastics school, the theater, piano lessons, and the charitable foundation we serve, sharing a passion with fellow patients, gym buddies, parents, adult piano students and foundation volunteers. Time with each of these tribes has grown since retirement and has given me more freedom to create new roles and a new sense of usefulness.

Finding my new element was relatively easy. I am lucky. Whether disabled or not, many people are not so lucky. Ken Robinson has a book for those disabled or non-disabled persons who have a harder time finding their element or their tribe. In Finding Your Element Robinson takes the reader through a process of reflection upon her/his life, imagining possibilities and ultimately discovering what the reader's own element probably is and where the reader's tribe might be found.

Summary

Disability is just one of the life events that can dramatically change what a person can do. A life with purpose and meaning may be suddenly gone. I found it important to live in the present with my disability. With few glances back at my former life, I considered what I loved to do as the person I had become. Now I spend time in my element every day.

I have reenlisted with some of the tribes I enjoyed before disability, developing a changed role and fresh commitment at the Los Niños de la Calle con Wendy Foundation and my gym. I have found new groups of like-minded people in my tribes at The Attic Theater, Complete Balance Solutions rehabilitation, and granddaughter Emma's gymnastics.   And I have found Ken Robinson is right when he teaches, "Discover your talents and passions and transform your life."

Notes

Ken Robinson's website has his writings and speeches available to browse. http://sirkenrobinson.com/

The Element by Ken Robinson is the foundation to all of Ken Robinson's writings and TED presentation. Here the concept of The Element and The Tribe that I use in this chapter are first introduced.

Finding Your Element: *How to find your element and tribe*

The Element: How Finding Your Passion Changes Everything by Ken Robinson includes stories about many famous people.

Finding Your Element by Ken Robinson is very useful for any disabled or non-disabled person needing to find his/her element.

Ken Robinson's first presentation at TED has been viewed more times than any other speaker's at TED ever. https://www.ted.com/talks/ken_robinson_says_schools_kill_cre ativity#t-912238

Ted.com has an easily accessible listing of their speakers who range from former Presidents to Nobel laureates, to masters of industry and beyond. Geniuses, artists and experts you will enjoy. With each presentation limited to 18 minutes, you often get a quick glimpse into a great (or simply interesting) person's work in one short sitting. Check out the TED channel on YouTube. You will see many of the live presentations and some related films as well.

Service
How serving others makes rehabilitation worthwhile

My life before spinal cord surgery was useful. I helped students learn at school, gave children's sermons at our church, wrote/directed Christmas pageants, volunteered in the Los Niños de la Calle con Wendy Foundation, regularly donated blood/platelets and kept my mouth shut when someone walked by wearing a New York Yankees shirt. Whatever I was ashamed of in my life and whatever guilt I felt for having so much good fortune, I was compensating for it in all sorts of ways. Or maybe I was just enjoying myself. I loved my job, directing/ writing plays and supporting the Foundation's good work. Even giving blood and platelets can be fun if you bring along DVDs to watch. Being useful was only difficult when I kept myself from bringing up the 2004 playoffs to a passing Yankee fan.

Lying in a bed at Cedars-Sinai Medical Center I did not feel useful anymore. I was a burden to Lynn, a patient the doctors could not fix and a helper who had fallen by the wayside, failing all the children and organizations I used to serve. When a phone call to my hospital room from a stressed colleague gave me the chance to counsel and encourage someone else, I began to be useful again. Returning to meaningful service had three benefits:

1. Those I served had better lives in some way.
2. I did not see myself as a useless cripple.
3. The possibility of providing more and greater service motivated me to get stronger.

Foundation
The Los Niños de la Calle con Wendy Foundation was founded in 2005 in memory of Wendy Trujillo, a fifth grade teacher I had recruited to join the faculty of Kaiser Elementary School. The school was more than twenty per cent Hispanic and the faculty was zero per cent Hispanic when I took over as principal. Wendy was an intelligent bilingual Hispanic teacher destined to advance into the still too meager ranks of Hispanic school administrators when she died in a car accident.

Service: *How serving others makes rehabilitation worthwhile*

Using a few hundred dollars in memorial contributions, her family started a foundation which continues to this day. Her father Jose Trujillo, a room service waiter at a Disneyland hotel, has done a better job of running a charitable foundation than anyone I have encountered in the nonprofit world. In 2015, continuing a pattern sustained every year since it began, the Foundation served meals to homeless persons at two Anaheim parks every Sunday, provided one thousand back packs filled with school supplies to poor students, awarded scholarships to high school seniors with outstanding community service records, donated clothing to an orphanage in Tijuana, Mexico, and provided food baskets to families in crisis both in Mexico and California.

Using my wheelchair or scooter I helped out in small ways. While other Foundation volunteers served a meal to hundreds of homeless persons in a large church activities hall, I handed out soap, toothpaste and shampoo to those who would use the showers and bathrooms. I sold raffle, game and meal tickets to the wonderful people who came out to our fundraising picnic.

It did not feel like I was as much help as I had been before the tumor at these events, so it really lifted me to find ways to help in ways that other volunteers could not. I took over the bookkeeping and annual filings with the IRS and California Franchise Tax Board as well as the annual re-registration as a 501c(3) charitable foundation. Churning administrative paperwork in the virtual back office of the Foundation has become a unique and important service I can accomplish whether my legs are having a good day or not.

Family

In 2016 Lynn told me how she remembers 2010 and 2011, the years of surgery, hospitalization and early rehabilitation. She remembers trying to think of everything I was going to need from moment to moment. She hurriedly made our new home wheelchair accessible while also shuttling to be with me in the hospital every day. Once I was home, she was my chauffeur to doctors, radiation treatments, physical therapy and my return to work. She hovered anxiously over every transfer I made from chair to wheelchair to toilet to bed to shower to car. The "new normal" as she put it then was taking over her whole life. Time and energy to be grandma, to work on her many projects and to enjoy her retirement were all lost to my needs. My stubborn pursuit of independence for the next five years freed her from that total dedication. "Thank you," she said looking back five years later, "for giving me my life back."

Many of my rehabilitation goals focus on what I can do to help more at home. I recall the first time I could take the trash cans to the curb. I controlled my scooter with one hand and pushed the trashcan with the other. Later I could use a walker and then a cane. In 2015 I made the trip to the road just using the trashcan itself for balance for the first time. The walk back up the driveway without the trashcan "walker" is a challenge, but I make it every week for the trash, recycling and green waste pickups. I am proud to be able to unload fifty-pound bags of soil and mulch after a trip to the garden center. I can cook, do dishes and maneuver around the kitchen confidently. I have progressed from a scary transfer from wheel chair to shower chair with Lynn anxiously standing by to independent showering without a shower chair both at home and in the locker rooms at gyms. I shop for all the items Lynn has texted to me at the grocery store, pharmacy and other shops while getting some exercise for my legs.

As I close in on my first 100,000 miles of driving with hand controls, I am a confident taxi driver for our three nearby grandchildren who need rides home from school as well as to and from sports practices / competitions, part-time jobs and play time with friends.

Advocacy

I have acted as the spokesperson for our Foundation in the struggle to provide permanent shelter for homeless individuals. Believe it or not, Orange County California, home to the third highest number of millionaires of all the counties in America, still has no permanent homeless shelter. I have been able to provide written testimony in many cases and testified in person a few times. After decades of public school board meetings, I am comfortable presenting before public bodies. Happily, we are making progress. A shelter for homeless people in Orange County has been approved.

I have helped get the vote out by working the phones in the weeks before elections. My values and beliefs become part of a campaign with texts, phone calls and letters. No matter that it's not easy for me to knock on doors anymore; I can influence hundreds of voters in critical areas all over the country with just a telephone.

The American with Disabilities Act (ADA), along with other state and federal statutes and accompanying regulations, is meant to guarantee persons with disabilities reasonable accommodations, such as handicap designated parking spaces, grab bars in rest rooms, ramps and elevators. The law is enforced by municipal and higher level code enforcement officers to some extent, but most of the enforcement is left to the disabled persons themselves. Access to courts and enforcement bureaus is relatively easy. In California, complaints can be brought in small claims court for a filing fee of $50. Federal ADA suits can be filed electronically for no initial fee.

I overlooked many ADA violations I encountered in the first years after my tumor surgery. I complained to some business owners who improved their practices. Finally I hit a few situations where I had to get formal and file. It was hard to take action; I did not relish the return to adversarial encounters. But I had started to feel a sense of obligation to the many disabled persons who cannot file actions. After all, the legislature pretty much left ADA enforcement to the disabled themselves. I have won some cases and settled others. No judge has ruled against me; my cases have always been worthy.

Some believe those of us who sometimes file ADA lawsuits are a bigger problem than ADA scoff-laws. Everyone did not support my action against a business that would not even talk to me about their selling clothing from racks set up in their handicap parking spaces and failing to provide handicap accessible rest rooms, among other ADA violations. Instead, the business hired a lawyer to bully me. An ADA suit is an unpleasant last resort, but this business, like others, was not willing to acknowledge its law breaking and make a commitment to improve until they were twenty feet from the courtroom door and on the docket for trial within the next hour. When they finally offered to improve their practices, I readily agreed to their settlement offer. If that makes me a litigious old crank, so be it. The world needs more cranks and fewer enablers anyway.

Church

I returned to church work soon after coming home from the hospital. I remember my first children's sermon. The scene of a strong church friend helping me to the front of the church made the children wary. But with some encouragement from their parents they came forward and sat around me, as was the custom in that church. It felt good to be able to resume many of the roles I had in the church, including weekly men's Bible study sessions, just about every Sunday worship service and some Elder meetings.

School

After surgery I was able to return to service as a school principal. I completed the second semester of the year and retired to focus more completely on rehabilitation. I am glad my career in education ended that way. Combining work and outpatient rehabilitation was difficult, but it bolstered those first months after the hospital to be able to return to my life's work and leave my profession with time to say good-byes and enjoy some of the final moments with my students, their families and of my co-workers. I still advise and counsel colleagues from time to time. I would undertake on line teaching, consulting or perhaps some other roles if the right opportunity should come along. The schoolhouse door is closed right now, but perhaps not forever.

Summary

Disabled persons serve others for three important reasons: First, there are family members and friends who need the disabled person's help. Others in the community and beyond can be lifted with even small acts of caring. Second, service provides a disabled person a useful role in life. And third, sustaining and building one's ability and capacity to serve is powerful motivation for rehabilitation.

In 2016 Lynn had surgery to relieve the spinal stenosis that caused pinched nerves in her neck and radiating pain down her right arm. The day after surgery she was sent home with a supply of heavy-duty pain pills. A day later, she woke up after a long nap in our family room needing to get to the bathroom quickly but feeling a little unsteady from the deep sleep and the heavy haze of all the medications. She asked me to walk with her, so that she could get to the bathroom safely. That's right, she asked me, the paraplegic. I never willed my spastic legs to behave themselves more than I did for those few steps down the hall. I was like a rock as Lynn leaned heavily on my arm. As she closed the door and left me out in the hall, I tearfully thanked every therapist who ever worked with me. Every struggle to lift an exhausted leg in the gym just one more time for the past five years was absolutely worth it. I was able to serve.

Notes
Los Niños de la Calle con Wendy. http://fundacionwendy.org/

Filing a federal ADA claim on line is simple. All you need to get started is at http://www.ada.gov/filing_complaint.htm. California ADA claims are easiest through the Small Claims Courts. http://www.disabilityrightsca.org/pubs/520601.pdf

Bucket List
How disability is a chance to accomplish lifelong dreams

Bucket List is a Rob Reiner directed film with Morgan Freeman and Jack Nicholson portraying two men coming to terms with terminal disease. They each write a "bucket list" of things they want to do before they kick the bucket. They decide to do as many of those things as they can in the time they have left. Two men who meet as roommates in a hospital room become friends and fellow adventurers.

I was surprised to encounter much younger people using the same expression. Actors in their early middle age have told me they were auditioning for a show I was directing, because that show was on their personal bucket lists. Disability is usually not as traumatic a diagnosis as terminal disease, but it ranks up there with retirement, death of a loved one, divorce, losing a job and relocation as a time when one takes stock of what has happened so far in life and what is yet to come.

There are two huge risks in this process. One can look back to what might have been if the disability had never happened and get lost in the past. Disability does not give us the past to relive, nothing does. But it does give us a different life to live, albeit a life with some major inconveniences. Those inconveniences are the other risk. In dealing with them, one can get lost in the parade of doctor visits, medications, rehab sessions and medical research. Working hard at rehab must not become obsession or escape.

The risks aside, disability does give us the opportunity, indeed the obligation, to reinvent our lives. Beyond the looking back and after all the time it takes to deal with the disability itself every day, there is something a disabled person may never have enjoyed before. Time. Time no longer consumed by a job, tending to others and whatever else filled our lives before disability.

This is not the time discussed in other chapters to manage one's disability using Jim Collins' school bus metaphor or to find a new life's work using Ken Robinson's concepts of the element and the tribe or even to discover a more playful life with an attitude of one's own choice following the FISH! Philosophy. This is not even the time needed for strategic breaks to meditate, enjoy a massage or a movie night, so that you are ready to go back at your recovery again afterward.

This chapter is about the time to do what we want, maybe for no particular purpose at all. Think of when your parents asked what you had been doing all afternoon and you said, "Nothing" just to keep them from intruding on your private joy with toys, reading, daydreaming, drawing or whatever. Or think of what came to mind when you took a break in the work day and imagined what you would do if you did not have to go back to finish that day at work or maybe never go back to that job at all.

My Bucket List:

- *Baseball.* Games I used to catch just in pieces on the radio driving home from work, I can now watch as much as I want. Being able to watch one show on television with Lynn while a baseball game is playing on my laptop is wonderful. My school schedule no longer controls when I can take a road trip to see the Red Sox play in Phoenix, San Diego, Anaheim, Los Angeles, Oakland or San Francisco. We have even flown up to Seattle; Lynn has high school friends to visit on an island northwest of Seattle. Our 2012 trip to spring training in Florida was our first March vacation ever. We got to see great friends from my years as Superintendent in Little Ferry, New Jersey. Joan and Joe Rizzo are basking in their Florida retirement far from the Garden State's howling blizzards.
- *Theater.* Most of my years in school administration included so many night meetings that I could not make it to rehearsals or performances for community theater. In an unusually good year I squeezed in just one show. Now I have found time for as many as three shows in a year. I sit on the Board of Directors for the Attic Theater. Lynn has been able to do some of the recent shows with me. (The only thing better than a flexible calendar is two flexible calendars.)
- *Movies.* We see more theater, concerts and movies than we ever could before my disability. We see most movies at home

and have become much more versed in good television, making use of all the recording functions to have our favorites all cued up and ready to watch. Disability shortens my day. Whoever said doing something with a spinal cord injury is seven times as hard as doing the same thing without a SCI is right. At the end of most days, I am usually ready to relax in front of the television.

- *Travel.* A separate chapter describes our travel since my disability. From the bucket list perspective, we found the time to go off on adventures, family visits and discoveries after our schedule opened up. Moreover, travel became fun, not the hectic hassle of business travel.

- *Friends.* I do Facebook by proxy. Lynn catches me up with FB every morning as she looks through our friends' postings. I

> A friend is someone who understands your past, believes in your future, and accepts you today just the way you are.
>
> Proverbs 17:17

maintain a LinkedIn account and see a few colleagues there. My CaringBridge blog keeps me current with more friends. We hang out, entertain, visit and do things together with our neighbors, theater friends, school friends, fellow foundation volunteers, and families of our grandkids' friends.

- *Grandkids.* I have worked with Kyle on college planning, scholarship applications and test preparation. Lynn and I both taxi Kyle, Amanda and Emma to sports, friends, work, haircuts, doctors and shopping. Each of the local grandkids has learned gardening, cooking, manners, family history and much more from time with grandparents. Grandma and Grandpa have learned even more. For the faraway grandkids, we are freer to travel when they are off from school or taking some family vacation time.

- *Projects.* Lynn has completed one project after another to upgrade, expand and beautify our houses and yards since we have been together. Seven houses in all. Now that my job obligations have ended, I have been able to help as my rehabilitation has progressed.

- *Romance.* During the years of our high-powered careers there was rarely a day when we did not speak on the phone. We might have been in different time zones, but we connected. One year, I was working in New York and commuting home to Michigan every weekend. Another year I was working in Michigan and commuting home to California every weekend. Many years, Lynn was off to the airport on Monday or Tuesday and back home Thursday or Friday. Since I came home from tumor surgery in 2010, we have said good night to each other by phone only three times. Lynn visited Brian and his family in Kentucky by herself and each of us has had a one-night stay in the hospital. Disability has brought together at last two love-struck kids who can leave their phones untouched on their night tables from now on.

Summary

I was fortunate to be cast as Grandpa in the Attic Theater's production of You Can't Take It with You. Grandpa has been retired for 35 years when the play starts. He had a successful business career going when he just walked out. In Act III, he gets into an argument with a man about his age who stayed with his business career and thinks Grandpa is irresponsible, or worse. Grandpa describes his retirement with this speech:

> Well, I have a lot of fun. Time enough for everything – read, talk, visit the zoo now and then, practice my darts, even have time to notice when spring comes around. Don't see anybody I don't want to, don't have six hours of things I have to do every day before I get one hour to do what I like…. I used to go down to that office nine o'clock sharp no matter how I felt. Lay awake nights for fear I wouldn't get that contract…. What I'm try to say is that I've had thirty-five years that nobody can take away from me, no matter what they do to the world….. [Moss Hart & George S. Kaufman, You Can't Take It with You.]

Whether disability takes one into retirement or into some other phase of life, it is an event we can use to discover time to visit the zoo, watch baseball or whatever joys have been crowded out. Once we put aside leftovers from our able-bodied life and avoid the trap of over-focus on the disability itself, there is an opportunity to (re)make a bucket list and enjoy the chance to check off some of the great experiences on the list. As Jack Nicholson and Morgan Freeman portrayed so poignantly, it turns out that the list is not so important as the adventures pursuing it.

Notes
Bucket List trailer:
https://www.youtube.com/watch?v=vc3mkG21ob4

You Can't Take It With You has more than a great speech in it. It's funny and entertaining. The family portrayed can give any of us, disabled or not, much to think about. They fill their lives with the things they enjoy. The movie has been made more than once and the play remains a staple of community theaters everywhere and occasional Broadway revivals. The TV revival with Jason Robards trailer:
https://www.youtube.com/watch?v=mzuKHNvPThw
The Best Picture Oscar winning 1938 film (Lionel Barrymore, Jimmy Stewart) trailer:
https://www.youtube.com/watch?v=0WY9RAroTS0
A montage from the 2014 Broadway revival:
https://www.youtube.com/watch?v=7cVkCnN7k3I

Remember, all of the internet sites in this book can be reached through http://tinyurl.com/StacyHolmesAuthor. You will not have to type in each site I like in the book. Go to this one site and you can easily click on any site mentioned in this book.

Travel
How travel rewards and motivates rehabilitation

My world after disability started with a gurney. I could not even roll over without help. Legs that had moved for 61 years to flip my weight onto one hip, the other hip, my back or belly just lay there inertly. The edge of the bed was the end of my world. Before I left the hospital a month later my world was larger. I could get into a wheelchair on my own, get to the elevator and buy some ice cream at one of the hospital shops.

That much mobility got me to the parking garage. I had learned how to open a car door while still in my wheel chair, use my upper body to pull myself upright using the car door as a support, turn away from the open door, find the car seat behind me with my hand, then lower myself into the seat using one hand on the door and the other on the seat to control the descent. I could not feel the seat with my butt. The sensation of weight further up my spine told me I was on the car seat and I could slowly relax my grip on the car door. After I lifted my legs with my hands into the car, I was ready for my world to get even bigger.

Road Trips
Our first road trip was from the hospital to home. Los Angeles to Mission Viejo, 63 miles of southern California freeways. I was thrilled to be out of the hospital and more thrilled to be with Lynn all the time instead of just during her daily visits to the hospital. We had never slept apart for a month. But the speed of the cars in five or more lanes each way scared me. Only a month away from the highways, and I had forgotten the speed of the outside world.

A few months later, we were enjoying a wider world a few times each year, and I was doing most of the driving on those crowded speedways. We were motivated by family gatherings for the most part, but we enjoyed the change of scenery and routine as well. My world no longer ended at the edge of the bed. Instead, I still got cabin fever with the routines of therapy and limitations of movement. Road trips were adventures, vacations from routines and welcome distractions. Places I knew as an able bodied person I would get to know all over again as a disabled person.

Tucson

Sister-in-law (and greatly esteemed editor of this book) Merrilee has lived in Tucson for 21years. She was the nearest family for my parents during their Tucson retirement years. (Dad died in Tucson. Mom moved back to Holmes farm country in New Hampshire after that.) Merrilee retired from the University of Arizona's business school. Tucson has spectacular weather with many open space natural parks, museums and trails that are readily accessible by wheelchair. A university town, its academic and professional theaters have provided many great nights of entertainment for us. Their directors and performers range from developing college theater students to professionals who have semi-retired in Tucson after careers on the stage or in film. We have attended the Tucson Festival of Books. It's held on the large University of Arizona campus, so a mobility scooter is a better idea than a wheelchair. We enjoyed presentations and Q&A sessions with best-selling authors. Restaurants and shopping are all roll-up easy in Tucson, running the gamut from bodega shops to large indoor malls. Much of the Native American and Hispanic culture is celebrated in Tucson's cuisine, art, architecture, apparel and performances. Venues large and small welcome visitors. Tucson's large retirement community obliges everyone welcoming customers, visitors or audiences to make sure their facilities are accessible.

Tucson is a 90-minute drive from Phoenix, hub of Major League Baseball's Cactus League, the spring training home of many professional teams. The Red Sox spring training is in Florida now; they did their spring training in Arizona when I was a boy. "Cactus League" was a sports term I remember from early childhood. Merrilee took us to a Cleveland Indians spring training game featuring Terry Francona, former Red Sox manager now doing the same job for the Indians.

Travel: *How travel rewards and motivates rehabilitation*

We reach Tucson in a day's driving. One of the routes is more picturesque with desert landscapes that make us think we are visiting another planet. There is some elevation on the route, and once we had to remember our New England driving skills when we met a snow storm in the mountain passes. (Later that same day, we were happily arrived in Tucson enjoying the sunshine in shorts and tee shirts.)

Sacramento

I have lived in states with dreary capital cities like Trenton, New Jersey or charming small town capitals like Montpelier, Vermont. Boston is my favorite city in the world, but its status as Massachusetts state capital hardly reaches my perception. Getting to know California, I expected Sacramento might be a dull, big state government town much like Albany, New York. But more like Boston, Sacramento has many attractions that have nothing to do with state government.

My first trips were to statewide school meetings and training sessions when I was still able bodied. Sacramento has an airport that is just big enough to attract major airlines, rental car companies and restaurants. I love that stage of a city's development before the airport becomes huge, a long way from downtown and time-consuming.

Sacramento is a city of trees. Even rundown neighborhoods have beautiful trees lining their streets. Trolley cars add character to the downtown. I have not tested their handicap accessibility but it's wonderful to see available and safe public transportation. Mass transit in California cities is far behind what is available in most American cities. Sacramento and San Francisco are catching up; southern California is a century behind.

Sacramento seems to me more of a kid town than government town. Restaurants with interesting cuisines mix with plain food eateries, sports bars and clubs in a midtown that has an active nightlife. 20-somethings and 30-somethings enjoy their city and each other after hours.

Emily took her residency for her first year after veterinary college at a Sacramento hospital. She stayed in the area another year so that her fiancé could finish up at University of California Davis. Steve plans on graduate school, so we may get introduced to another city if he goes someplace other than UC Davis for his doctorate.

Sacramento is seven hours from our home in Mission Viejo. Road trips have helped me stretch the time I can sit in a car. With a couple half-hour stops that include walking and stretching, Lynn's sciatica and my spastic legs make it more or less comfortably. Driving with hand controls, your feet must be well away from the pedals, so that they do not accidentally hit one of them. My right foot curls almost under my seat; after every three hours of driving, I need to give my leg and hip a break.

The shortest route takes us up through the central valley where so much of America's food is grown. Smelly vegetables (garlic) and factory-style dairy farms are not my favorite parts of the trip, but it always interests me to get through the mountains north of Los Angeles into farm country. There is so much of it, however, that the trip requires an interesting audio book.

We make the return trip via San Francisco (Lynn's brother Jim, wife Dana and daughter Kit), San Jose (Jim's son Justin and family) and San Luis Obispo (Jim's son Ian). It is longer but much more interesting; we add one or two overnights to give us time to visit. Jim, Dana and Kit live on a houseboat, giving me challenges to cane walk over floating piers and climb up a ladder to the houseboat's top deck. Nice to have all my hard work gaining balance and strength pay off by giving me access to fun adventures. These trips have also built my confidence at finding accessible hotels and figuring out how to get a good workout in their exercise rooms.

San Diego
I first visited San Diego in 1967. A rebel from my family's Ivy League / Seven Sister college tradition, I attended Antioch College, a liberal work/study college in Ohio. One of my work quarters was as a teacher aide at Camp Palomar. Each week a new load of sixth graders would bus up the mountain to visit the Palomar Observatory, hike through pristine state and national

wilderness areas and carve something out of the local Manzanita wood or alabaster stone to take home. Weekends I was on my own in San Diego. A Navy town, it was fun to get to the beach, the world famous zoo and the theaters. It was then and still is a city with areas you can enjoy on foot or scooter.

Coronado Island is right next to the city. I crutch walked out on the Coronado state beach one beautiful morning a couple years into my recovery to perform the marriage ceremony for my massage therapist Ernie and his wife Mary Beth. Lynn and I have stayed at the Coronado Marriott and enjoyed the quiet resort-like ambiance. You might imagine you are at an island

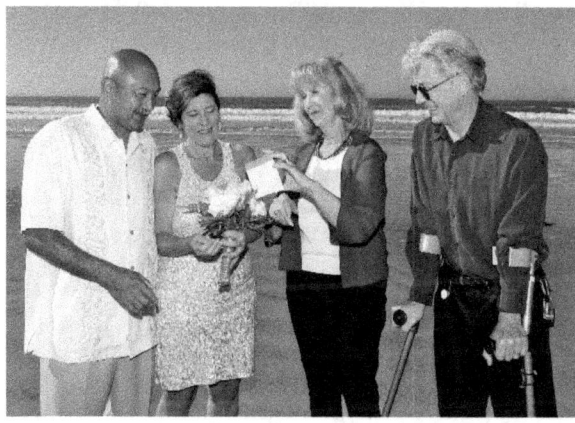

resort in the middle of nowhere, yet just a few minutes away stands the bridge back to San Diego with its theaters, sports stadiums and convention center. Few cities or resorts have that combination.

The Globe Theater in Balboa Park is a complex of stages with edgier works on the smaller stages and more mainstream productions on the large one. I had no trouble with access. Shows that have originated in The Globe and gone on to Broadway have won 9 Tonys and 60 nominations.

The San Diego Padres host the Boston Red Sox once every three seasons or so in their wonderful ballpark. We stay at a Marriott at the edge of the Gaslamp Quarter and walk and roll (some couples "rock and roll"; we "walk and roll") to the game. Not many games get rained out in San Diego. Bring sunscreen. I would not bring young students or grandchildren to some of the major league sports venues in baseball, football, basketball and hockey. The fan behavior and management are not suitable for children. San Diego is delightfully retro. Lots of kids enjoy the game in a family friendly stadium and culture.

Travel: *How travel rewards and motivates rehabilitation*

The 2015 State Meet for gymnastics was held in San Diego. It was eight-year-old Emma's first year in competitive gymnastics. We stayed at the convention center hotel, which again allowed us to "walk and roll" to the event. There were wide eyes that weekend. Emma was dazzled by her first visit to a large downtown hotel. Grandma and Grandpa as well as her whole family were amazed when she won second place all-around for the Level 3 eight-year-olds.

San Diego is a one- or two-hour drive from our home in Mission Viejo, depending on traffic. Much of the drive is close enough to the ocean to provide spectacular views. We like to consult those who make the trip more often than we do. Everyone seems to have a favorite restaurant somewhere along the way. There are also outlet shopping centers and amazing beaches en route.

Temecula

Our first wine tasting tour in California was Napa Valley and nearby Sonoma. Michigan friends Lynne and Don Wheaton shared some recommendations and even got us invited to a vineyard not normally open to the public. It is a nice added attraction to a San Francisco trip, but Napa has become too popular with the 1%. Prices have shot up and it has become a scene we do not enjoy as much anymore. We have not been back to Napa since my disability, but from my memory of our earlier trips, I would worry about some of the small vineyards' handicap access. And the small vineyards are often the most charming and interesting. It is hard to feel personally welcomed at a vineyard, or anywhere else, with three tour buses parked in front.

It turns out grapes grow almost anywhere in California. Only an hour and a half from home is Temecula, a rapidly growing community for year round and vacation homes. South Coast Winery Resort and Spa (a curious name for a spot in the high desert far from the coast) is a favorite stop for us. Wonderful spa treatments and facilities, a great restaurant and wines from moderate to expensive. The vineyards come right up to the windows of the hacienda style rooms. Their handicap accessible rooms are spacious, making it easy to maneuver a wheel chair anywhere. Pools, special event areas, the spa and grounds are easy with a wheel chair.

Exiting I-15 for Rancho California Road takes eager wine enthusiasts past at least a dozen vineyards of varying sizes and specialties. They are generally more handicap accessible than Napa and often include small or large restaurants with their tasting rooms. But do not miss Temecula Old Town. Some delightful local art and culture can be found in little independent shops mixed with the more touristy ice cream, candy, souvenir and coffee sellers. We found outstanding French bakeries for breakfast; Laurent's French toast made from croissants is a personal favorite. If you are not vegetarian, the cowboy restaurants are fun. Otherwise, gourmands will enjoy the variety of specialties featured by restaurants all along the main drag in Old Temecula. Usually side street parking is available. We parked and reparked as we explored, so that I could stay on crutches. The sidewalks are doable for longer treks by scooter with no need to find more parking. Temecula goes to sleep early. You will not find many places open for late night partying.

Flights
Road trips from overnight to a few days away built our skills and confidence for longer trips by airplane. I still look forward to the day that I can manage an airport without my scooter, but my cane or crutch walking limits are realistically about 45 minutes and a half mile. Anyone who flies knows you can easily encounter longer times and distances getting through large airports. Standing in line for even a few minutes is much harder on my legs than walking.

Boston
We have most frequently flown to Boston. Jet Blue has good service out of Long Beach, sometimes better service out of Los Angeles, but we avoid LAX if we can. It is further from our home, frequently tied up with security issues and always teeming with many thousands of travelers. Nonstop return flights are usually available, but we connect through Las Vegas going outbound to Boston. Long Beach is perhaps the easiest airport for handicap

access that I have found so far with the caveat that they do not have jet bridges. They will push your wheelchair up the ramps from the tarmac to the aircraft door. I gate check my scooter at the foot of the ramp and walk up using the sides of the ramps like the parallel bars at the rehab clinic to hold me up. They do a great job pushing you up the ramps in a wheel chair too.

Restrooms on airplanes changed from impossible to doable between year two and year four of my recovery. At first, I would stop eating and drinking a few hours before our flight, so that I would not have to use the restroom. Next, Lynn or a flight attendant walked backwards up the aisle to the restroom, so that I could grip her forearms while she gripped mine. Next were crutches on my own, but getting the crutches down from the overhead bin was a trick. Handicap passengers are boarded first; passengers boarding after us often put their baggage on top of my crutches. Finally, I just imitated the way flight attendants walk in rough weather using seat backs and overhead compartments for support. Now I can even take an extra moment to do a few stretches when I get up during our flights.

We stay with son Graham, his wife Jean and their daughters Megan and Lauren in their historic home in Medfield, Massachusetts, a Boston suburb. I scrambled up the stairs on all

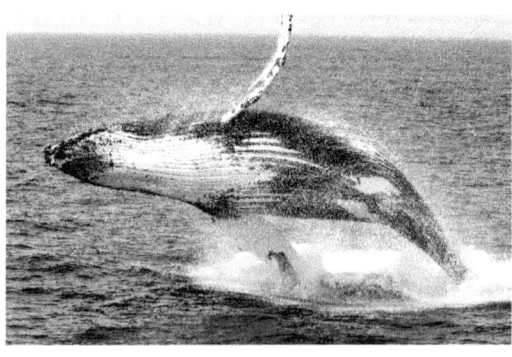

fours the first time we visited. Now I can walk up and down the stairs relying on Graham's handyman skills that reinforced every banister in the house. Our visits have let us enjoy Boston, Cape Cod and New England with easy day trips. We saw whales breaching one glorious afternoon. My brother Joe and his wife Eileen are two and a half hours north in Langdon, NH. We see them and overnight in Keene on most trips. Merrilee's daughter Lily, her husband Tim and their son Eddy were in Boston for all of our visits for the first five years of my recovery. Lily was a surgeon at Mass General before moving on to a post in Minnesota.

Fenway Park
Perhaps my greatest rediscovery of a familiar place from my able bodied days to my current mobility strategies was Boston's Fenway Park. Much as I love the old ball field, I could not imagine returning there as a disabled fan.

For more than a century, Fenway Park has been home for the Boston Red Sox. Now the oldest active stadium in major league baseball, Fenway Park is downtown in the midst of twisting little streets laid out (according to legend) on colonial cow paths. Fenway's most famous feature is the Green Monster – at 37 feet the highest outfield fence in baseball.

After my family moved from El Paso, Texas, where I was born, I grew from eight to fifteen years old on the small farm my family owned in Chelmsford, Massachusetts. My dad took our family to Fenway Park every summer. He would finesse the notorious Boston traffic and magically find the last parking spot on Commonwealth Avenue. Then he walked so fast I had to jog to keep up all the way to Fenway. Later, with graduate school and jobs in New England, I returned many times to Fenway Park with Dad (still straining to keep up with his walking). He never loved my hero Carl Yastrzemski as much as his own idol, Ted Williams. A newborn when the Red Sox won the World Series in 1918, Dad passed away just before the next time his team won the World Series in 2004. The three times the Red Sox have won it since then left me yearning he could have seen his boys of summer in their time of glory.

Back in New England for the first time after my surgery, I called to check on handicap seats for the home games during our visit with Graham and family. The Red Sox were in the middle of multiple seasons with every home game sold out. I expected that my inquiry was many months too late. The box office representative said the team often has seats available for handicapped fans even just a few days before a game. I managed to secure a wheel chair spot, a companion seat next to me for

Travel: *How travel rewards and motivates rehabilitation*

Graham and even a pair of seats nearby for our daughter Emily and her boyfriend (later fiancé) Steve.

Access issues for Fenway Park start a half mile from the ballpark. Kenmore Square is the undersized confluence of a major inner belt parkway (Storrow Drive), the Massachusetts Turnpike, the T (Boston's excellent public transit system) and two of Boston's busiest streets (Commonwealth Avenue and Beacon Street). Graham weaved expertly through jammed pre-game traffic, but still pedestrians around us were making much faster progress through Kenmore Square than we were. It was more than an hour before the game, and the parking lots were already sold out. Casting my eyes about for options, I spied somebody pulling out of a handicapped parking spot.

With that good fortune we parked within a reasonable scooter ride to Fenway Park. My electric three-wheeler had never before encountered the cobblestones and inclines that make up the path to Fenway Park from Kenmore Square. I was grateful for my six-foot companions Graham and Steve. Cars jockeying through the congestion saw the tall guys with me on the crosswalks long before they saw me seated on a scooter. The nerves in my body that still worked complained mightily about the jarring over the rough walkways. But we made it. We were ready to answer the ultimate question of the day: Is this century-old ballpark really accessible?

I was stunned. Fenway Park seemed utterly inadaptable to disabled people as I had thought about it from my perspective of 40+ years as an able-bodied Sox fan. But I was so wrong. I went up a little ramp made of concrete that looked like part of the original 1910 construction. A walkway between the lower and upper grandstand seats had been widened. Perhaps they took out a row of seats to gain the added space. Able bodied fans easily crisscrossed the walkway behind the wheel chair fans and their companions enjoying the game. Amazing.

As the game progressed, I ventured on my own to the men's room and concessions. Without family members to run interference, I encountered the greatest accommodation any handicapped person can ask for in a public place – fantastic people. Fenway ushers directed me to the ramps and away from the steps. Rowdy, fun-loving guys hollered at their friends to get out of my way. I became part of their fun. Goofing around with fellow fans at Fenway Park, it was like old times.

There are stadiums and theaters I no longer try to access as I return to my beloved concerts, games and performances in a wheel chair or scooter. All of these rejected venues were constructed long after Fenway Park was built. The Red Sox organization did some ingenious engineering and adopted the right attitude to make their very old ballpark one of the most accommodating places I have visited anywhere. I cannot wait for my next game at Fenway Park.

Florida

My first full year of retirement was 2012. I felt like I had waited my entire career in education to be free to travel to Spring Training. Lynn and I used up the last of our Continental/ United Airlines frequent flier miles from all our business travel days and flew to Fort Meyers, Florida, home of Red Sox Spring Training. We arrived at midnight eastern time and found our Alamo rental car with hand controls shiny clean and with the trunk open to receive the scooter and luggage. Short drives from our hotel not only got us to Jet Blue Field at Fenway South but also to the spring training field of other teams, allowing us to see the Sox at home and on the road.

Florida is the escape from Northeast and Midwest winters for millions. Many stay a week while the kids are on school vacation, many others party for a little longer then go back to college when spring break is over and still more spend every winter for the rest of their retirement in the sunshine. Florida is also the first stop in America for many Cubans as well as a great many others from the Caribbean and Latin America. The abundant supply of service workers attend to the generous supply of vacationers and retirees. They also grow delicious oranges and launch a few space rockets.

I found the smaller ball parks used for spring training easier to manage just because they are smaller. Shorter distances from parking to stadium, entrance to seats, seats to restroom and concessions. Florida demographics have convinced restaurants, museums, hotels, bookstores, theaters and anywhere else you might visit that more access and better access is better business.

New York Finger Lakes

The Empire State has a great variety of water. In my 20s I canoed with Boy Scouts in the wilderness streams of the Adirondacks. I visited Niagara Falls, the St. Lawrence Seaway, the Hudson River valley, Lake George, Lake Placid Olympic village, Lake Erie and the Atlantic Ocean. In the middle of the state are the long and narrow Finger Lakes. Canadaigua, Seneca, Oswego, Cayuga, Owasco, Skaneateles, Otisco and Keuka Lakes lay beside each other like fingers.

We visited Aurora on Lake Cayuga to attend nephew Darwin's (sister Nancy's youngest son) and Ashley's marriage. We stayed in the Aurora Inn where the wedding was held. The 1833 Federalist style Inn has been upgraded in a manner that makes visitors feel they are visiting a museum as much as being pampered with four-star accommodations and service. The elevator and rest room grab bars made our room, the restaurant and all the common rooms accessible for me. Our room shared a balcony overlooking Main Street. Its sturdy rail became my hand hold for daily walking stints to keep my legs working. We enjoyed great lunches and breakfasts at the Inn and at nearby spots on Main Street. MacKenzie-Childs is nearby. Give yourself half a day to tour the museums, store, educational presentations and artisans' shops. Their furniture and furnishings are not our style and way out of our price range, but that does not diminish the fun. I had some tight turns on my scooter in some of the little houses they have made into museums to display their products, but I was able to see all of the public areas.

We chose to fly into New York and drive up to the Finger Lakes. Once out of New York City, it was a pleasant drive with lots of memories for us former New Englanders. Landing closer to Aurora would have meant a second flight; there is no direct service from any southern California airport to Syracuse. I am not sure we made the right choice. Changing planes to another airline is a hassle, but the city driving was not much fun either.

Travel: *How travel rewards and motivates rehabilitation*

Tenants Harbor, Maine

By summer of 2015 we had become bolder in our adventures. We split the rental of a house in Tenants Harbor, Maine with Graham and Jean. We had a wonderful time with granddaughters Megan and Lauren. The ocean waves were broken further out by the coves and islands along that area of the Maine coast, but the tidal flow at high tide brought water right up to the edge of the trees lining the back of the rental property. With Graham's strong arm for support, I was able to get into a kayak (very ungracefully). Graham and I were a hapless comedy team trying to steer a two-man kayak, but we did very well in two solo kayaks. It was a new accomplishment in my independence, wonderful exercise and a unique way to sight see on the Maine coast. We savored homemade ice cream at a roadside stand, fresh-caught seafood and a lobster dinner cooked by Graham and Jean. There were local artists exhibiting in shops and their own homes. We viewed Fourth of July fireworks from a high spot that allowed us to see three different nearby towns firing off their skyrockets at the same time. On the drive back to Graham and Jean's home, we stopped at L.L.Bean in Freeport, Maine. Located in an outdoor mall with a dozen other outlet style stores, the home base of the New England outfitter for rural life is a fun stop.

The Maine coast is a half-day drive north from Boston. Only a couple hours from suburban Boston, the scene shifts to a quieter, slower paced seascape. We stopped at random mom-and-pop road houses as well as places with great reviews on Yelp. All of them had easy accommodations for me and great food.

I have learned to relax when we pull up to some little place. True, the big chains have more standardized, predictable accommodations for disabled patrons. But I have learned that smaller places – being smaller -- have smaller access issues. Small places often have owners and loyal employees who take pride in their hospitality. Busy maitres-d'hotel in fancy restaurants might point the way to the men's room. A little place on the Maine roadside will have a local kid working there who will walk with me, offer a supporting arm, and fill me in on the local places to visit.

Summary

We have become confident travelers by carefully planning trips and realizing that we can make adjustments as we go along to avoid exhaustion, frustration or disappointment. Travel motivates my rehabilitation, so that I can do more on our next trip. The complete break from routine provides a fresh start when we return to the gyms and clinics back home. The internet provides many preview opportunities as well as direct contact to home rental agents and others who often make special preparations for disabled guests once we have gotten to know each other ahead of time by email.

Notes

South Coast Winery Resort and Spa:
http://www.southcoastwinery.com/

We have had consistently good service from Jet Blue and United. They have handled my scooter without damage and retrieved it promptly upon landing, so that we could head off to baggage claim with the rest of the passengers. We have not had good luck with Delta or Virgin America.

Alamo has provided excellent rental cars. Their hand control installations are the best of the rental cars I have driven. Enterprise has had mostly excellent service for us as well. A few lapses were handled well. They have refunded rentals when the car has not been ready on time. I will not go to Hertz again.

Smaller airports are almost always more handicap accessible than large ones. Long Beach, Sacramento, John Wayne (Orange County) and Fort Meyers tempt me to leave my scooter home because they require so little walking. Bush (Houston), JFK (New York) and O'Hare (Chicago) are difficult enough to be avoided. JFK's rental cars can be reached only via a non-handicap accessible bus. Fellow passengers had to load my scooter on the bus and lift me into it. Newark is the only NYC airport I will consider in the future. Logan (Boston) and San Francisco have the long distances of large international airports, but they have much more consistently thought out and provided handicap accessibility throughout their facilities.

A four minute video capturing the history of Fenway Park: https://www.youtube.com/watch?v=DyZnqCGDgh4 A few years ago the team built a new spring training facility that is the same size and shape as Fenway Park in Boston. Here are some views of the spring training ball park: https://www.youtube.com/watch?v=Y27RK1O-Jsk

More on the Aurora Inns at www.innsofaurora.com. The company has acquired, renovated and opened a number of inns, not just the Aurora Inn. All with fascinating histories and renovation tales.

MacKenzie-Childs is quite an experience on their website. http://www.mackenzie-childs.com/ If you get a chance to visit, you will be amazed. You will enjoy the backstage tour of production studios. Artisans make each piece individually. The displays range from educational tours / slideshows to a large retail store to several rooms and separate houses devoted to museum-style displays of their furniture and furnishings including both their current products and some sold earlier in the MacKenzie-Childs history.

Remember, all of the internet sites in this book can be reached through http://tinyurl.com/StacyHolmesAuthor. You will not have to type in each site I like in the book. Go to this one site and you can easily click on any site mentioned in this book.

Conclusion
How you will be part of my next book

As I finish writing this book, my one-day-at-a-time rehabilitation has reached 1,987 days. It would have been a shorter book if there were a simple way to keep at daily recovery. But, at one time or another, each of the perspectives of disability I've described kept me going. Whether you are dieting, getting back in shape, going on the wagon, quitting cigarettes, stopping drugs, ending an obsession, getting past a traumatic event, mending a serious injury or recovering from disease, you will discover, as I did, that some days:

- You review your disability history to give yourself credit for every little bit of progress.

- You forgive yourself for your sins of pride, lust, gluttony, sorrow, greed, anger and sloth if they help you get better.

- You try the next gadget, medication or technique that might help you.

- You discover ways to play at rehabilitation, include others in your fun and keep your focus on playful recovery by choosing your attitude.

- You give yourself a strategic rest to let your fried brains cool off and weary muscles recover.

- You manage the business of rehabilitation. You figure out who is needed on your rehabilitation bus trip and who should get off at the next stop.

- You create and enjoy the creations of others. Redecorating, listening to music, Facebooking, seeing a show, reading, sewing, videoing with your phone, writing, cartooning or any way you might find imaginary places, beautiful sights and thrilling experiences.

- You find what you can do as a disabled person that you love to do and can become good at doing. You connect with others in your tribe who share your element and passion.

- You help someone else. Being useful feels good and makes you want to get stronger to be even more useful.

- You plan out what you will enjoy doing with the time left in life. The planning itself is fun. Checking off the adventures on your bucket list is even better.

- You broaden your horizons by getting out of town to see people and places.

I hope this book has given you ideas for your life, whether you are disabled or temporarily able bodied. My spinal cord injury and your struggle may not be alike, but the perspectives needed for my long-term recovery and yours are much more alike. Check out the books, websites and YouTube videos I have gathered in the Notes sections. This book only skims the surface of so many useful resources. There is much more waiting for you if you take the time to delve more deeply into the ones that interest you.

Your Story – My Next Book
I have been educated, inspired and entertained by many disabled friends. We get stronger by doing our exercises and taking our medicines. Counselors, friends and family support our mental and spiritual recovery. But our tribe consists of our disabled brothers and sisters. We learn best from each other. My next book profiles disabled persons' rehabilitations.

Please email me at fenwayfever48@gmail.com to share your story or recommend someone else in a long term rehabilitation. I am excited to get our stories organized and published. There is so much more for all of us to learn from each other and so many great new friends to meet.

Appreciation
How family, friends, tribes and bus riders made this book

I am overcome with gratitude and admiration. The team that brought this book into existence is talented, loving and generous.

My sister **Rev. Nancy Nyberg** tutored me on the Amazon self-publishing process. She turned me on to Rick Smith's invaluable book on the topic. You may have discovered this book because I followed her

My sister-in-law **Merrilee Holmes** edited the manuscript masterfully. Her suggestions made every page of the book more readable and everything I have tried to communicate clearer.

My wife **Lynn Holmes** has also edited the manuscript, helped me develop the concepts, and taken most of the pictures. As she did with all that came before, she welcomed this latest rehabilitation project into our lives together with tender love and encouragement.

Stepson **Zachary Plonski** helped with the cover and made all the arrangement for the audio edition of this book. **Danny Willy** recorded and edited the audio book. **Grupo Gallegos Advertising Agency** opened their audio studio to me.

CaringBridge readers, theater friends, rehab friends and therapists encouraged me to write this book and cheered me in the process when I was finally able to revisit all these days and tell the story.

I have tried to verify facts and get permission to use images. If there are corrections I should make or images I should delete, please let me know, and I will make the changes at the first opportunity.

From the outset there were healers, tribe members and friends who jumped on my rehabilitation bus. They made my long-term rehabilitation possible. I am forever grateful to all of them as well:

Dr. Bruce Van Vranken has been my family doctor, guided my choices of specialists and kept the rest of my body healthy while the specialists battled with my tumor.

Dr. John Yu had the humility to realize my tumor resides where neurosurgeons cannot attack without devastating collateral damage. His choice to step back from the operating table at the right moment left me able to take up my life again. He has stayed on the case ever since making sure the tumor does not get up to any more mischief.

Dr. Srikanth Rao led the rehabilitation team at Cedars-Sinai that enabled me to go home safely and motivated me to continue in outpatient rehabilitation thereafter. He saw me as an outpatient for another two years, working with me to develop the medication protocol that continues to work today.

Christy Smitheran, co-owner of Precision Rehabilitation, got me into the right AFO leg braces and the right wheelchair. Her expertise specified the custom-made chair that I did not just sit in, but wore like a favorite pair of jeans for two years. She steered me to Ziad.

Dr. Ziad Dahdul is the Precision Rehabilitation physical therapist who worked with me two or three times a week for more than three years. He encouraged me to try moves I did not feel ready for, caught me when I messed up and entertained me with his expert sports analysis as we tried again. And again.

Dr. Mary Beth Pongetti is my current physical therapist at Complete Balance Solutions. The most academically accomplished PT I have met, she has found weak underperforming muscles hiding behind the efforts of stronger overworked ones. The clinic's focus on balance and Mary Beth's world-class analysis and therapy has created a new era of my rehabilitation.

Teddy Newsom has introduced me to music arrangers I enjoy and helped me learn many new piano pieces. Gaining the independence to get back to piano lessons on my own was an important objective for my first year of rehabilitation.

Ernie Villaneuva has worked on my body from before the tumor to now. He literally puts his finger on my improving strength, flexibility and sensation. His updates on my awakening nerves galvanize my determination to continue my rehabilitation.

Jim Huffman, co-owner of The Attic Theater, acted with me in my first show at his theater. He has performed in shows I have directed and created amazing scenery for every production. Jim has confidently assumed I would do well when I was inwardly fearful a role (acting or directing) was more than I could actually do. He is my second greatest cheerleader, and I hope I am his.

Jose Trujillo (President of Los Niños de la Calle con Wendy Foundation), his wife Margarita and their entire family have rushed to the hospital, helped in any way they could and continued to welcome Lynn and me into the Foundation's great work. If I wonder whether I am useful to anyone else after all the strength, energy and focus I have lost, Jose and his wonderful Foundation assure me there is still good work I can do.

These heroes sit in the front seats. Filling the rest of my rehab bus are members of the tribes who post encouraging notes on CaringBridge, FaceBook with Lynn, come see our shows at The Attic, sweat with me at the gym, persevere along with me at the rehab clinic, offer thumbs up as I toddle past them walking around the neighborhood – or take a few hours to read this book.

Thank you one and all.

www.ingramcontent.com/pod-product-compliance
Lightning Source LLC
Chambersburg PA
CBHW071155280526
45787CB00002B/506